# FINDING YOUR FIT

# FINDING YOUR FIT

## A Compassionate Trainer's Guide to Making Fitness a Lifelong Habit

## Kathleen Trotter

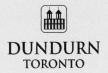

DUNDURN
TORONTO

Editor: Natalie Meditsky
Design: Courtney Horner
Cover design: Courtney Horner
Printer: Webcom
Cover photo by Malina Kaija

**Library and Archives Canada Cataloguing in Publication**

Trotter, Kathleen, author
Finding your fit : a compassionate trainer's guide to making fitness
a lifelong habit / Kathleen Trotter.

Issued in print and electronic formats.
ISBN 978-1-4597-3519-4 (paperback).--ISBN 978-1-4597-3520-0 (pdf).--
ISBN 978-1-4597-3521-7 (epub)

1. Health behavior.  2. Physical fitness.  3. Motivation (Psychology).
I. Title.

RA776.9.T76 2016                613.7                C2016-903877-7
                                                     C2016-903878-5

1   2   3   4   5        20   19   18   17   16

  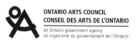

We acknowledge the support of the **Canada Council for the Arts** and the **Ontario Arts Council** for our publishing program. We also acknowledge the financial support of the **Government of Canada** through the **Canada Book Fund** and **Livres Canada Books**, and the **Government of Ontario** through the **Ontario Book Publishing Tax Credit** and the **Ontario Media Development Corporation**.

**VISIT US AT**
Dundurn.com | @dundurnpress | Facebook.com/dundurnpress | Pinterest.com/dundurnpress

Dundurn
3 Church Street, Suite 500
Toronto, Ontario, Canada
M5E 1M2

# CONTENTS

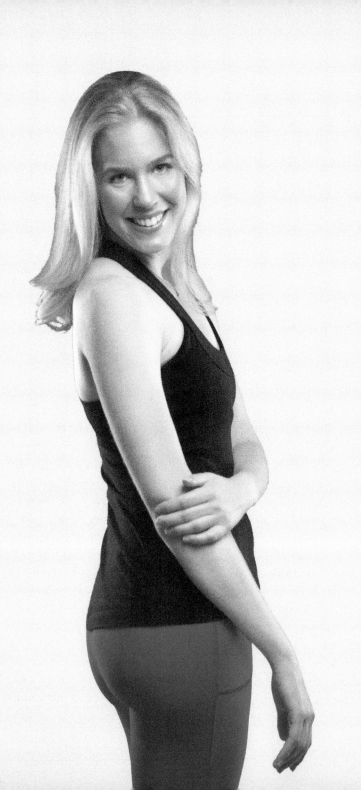

# INTRODUCTION

## My Story

Now that I'm an adult, I enjoy being six feet tall. I am proud of my body's capabilities; I love that I can run and that I am strong; that I can lift weights and compete in endurance events such as triathlons; and that when my family asks me to move furniture, I am as good as anyone at the job. As an adolescent, I definitely did not feel this way. I was chubby and awkward. I was taller and larger than everyone — including all the boys. I was sometimes even mistaken for a substitute teacher. I hated my body and had a microscopic level of self-esteem. I would do anything to get out of gym class. Even the idea of going to the locker room to change made me want to go home. I cried a lot and

often faked being sick in an attempt to be sent home. Not my proudest moments.

My life began to change roughly fifteen years ago when my mom bought me a membership to the YMCA. I started working out and taking exercise classes. Initially, my mom had to force me to go, but after the first couple of visits I didn't need much encouragement. I realized that I felt way more comfortable being active when I was surrounded by adults than I was in gym class with kids my own age. I gradually got to know everyone at the Y. It started to feel like a home away from home. I was young so my body adapted quickly. I lost weight and people started complimenting me, which gave me the incentive to keep

One of my goals as a trainer is to help initiate these positive domino effects. We all make hundreds of seemingly banal health choices. Instead of letting one less-than-ideal choice bleed into your mindset for the rest of the day, focus on the positive health choices you do make. Be proud of your positive choices, and let that pride inform your mindset and result in your own positive domino effect.

training. I started taking more and more classes, and eventually I took so many that the Y asked me to become an instructor. At first, putting my body on display in front of the twenty-or-so students in the class was petrifying, but I did it, and in time I learned to love being active, teaching, and motivating others. As an added bonus, my new-found physical awareness caused a positive domino effect: I started to become more aware of my nutritional choices and changed the way I was eating.

My mom always prepared healthy food, but I snuck unhealthy food. I used to tell my mom I wanted to walk home from school to get fresh air when really I just wanted to stop and buy fries at the chip wagon. An even more embarrassing story is that I would lie to cashiers about my junk food consumption. I would go the convenience store before school and buy Smarties (or m&m's or chocolate-covered almonds, or really anything chocolate — I have always been a sucker for chocolate). I would eat everything I bought and then go back to the convenience store at lunch and tell the cashier that I had spilled my Smarties (or my almonds) and

so I needed to buy more. I wanted another treat, but I felt guilty and ashamed about my weight and my eating choices, so I lied.

Gradually, as I got into being more active, I began to appreciate the importance of portion control, nutritious foods, and understanding why I was eating. Sure, I still have phases where I pay less attention to my diet, but I have never reverted back to being the girl who would lie to a cashier about spilling her Smarties.

The girl who would do anything to get out of gym class and was teased for "eating pasta with her cheese" now runs marathons, lifts weights, and (mostly) makes nutritious food choices. I aim to "own" all my health choices; when I want a treat, I mindfully and purposely enjoy a moderate portion of something I love (I call this my "love it" rule). I try not to feel guilt or let one piece of chocolate snowball into ten pieces of chocolate; I have one treat, not ten.

Joining the YMCA caused what I call my "positive health ripple." My hope is that this book will be your catalyst for change — the start of your positive health ripple. You too can own your choices.

# Your Health Journey Starts Today

Adopting a healthier lifestyle was the best thing that I ever did for myself. My outside appearance changed, but more important, my confidence and my energy increased. I became a personal trainer out of a desire to share the energizing and empowering nature of exercise with others — to help motivate everyone to learn to love and crave a healthier, more active lifestyle.

My goal is to motivate YOU — not only to adopt a healthier lifestyle, but to find a healthier lifestyle that you actually enjoy and can maintain for the rest of your life. I am sure you know that health is important (who doesn't?). You have probably even tried to make healthier choices multiple times, only to be derailed or discouraged and fall back into old habits. Don't worry, you are not alone. Most of us have participated in the health "on again, off again" cycle at least once or twice. The problem is, wanting to get on track and actually getting and staying on track are two totally different things.

Giving voice to what I call "fitness wishes" — such as "I want to get into shape" — is the easy part. Turning those wishes into long-term, sustainable, and safe fitness realities is harder.

There is no shortage of fitness books that offer the "complete" or "ultimate" workout, but no thirty-day fix will work if you never actually DO the program. The solution? Use the information in this book to put together a unique and realistic plan tailored to fit your individual lifestyle realities — what I refer to as "your recipe for success."

I started this chapter by laying out my personal health history. I did this to illustrate that I didn't form my current lifestyle overnight. I didn't flip a switch or wake up one morning a new person. Yes, getting the membership to the Y was a positive catalyst, but I still had to learn how to go to the gym regularly and enjoy moving. (I use learn purposely here; adopting a healthier lifestyle takes conscious thought and time. You have to learn and integrate new, healthier habits into your daily life.) Adopting a healthier lifestyle is a process — an active process. You have to be actively involved in forming the healthier version of yourself that you want to be.

Now, too many health and wellness products are sold on the promise of turning consumers into a whole new version of themselves overnight. I don't want to turn you into a whole new you. A "new you" implies that there is something wrong with the original version. Instead, I want you to learn to love yourself and value yourself. I

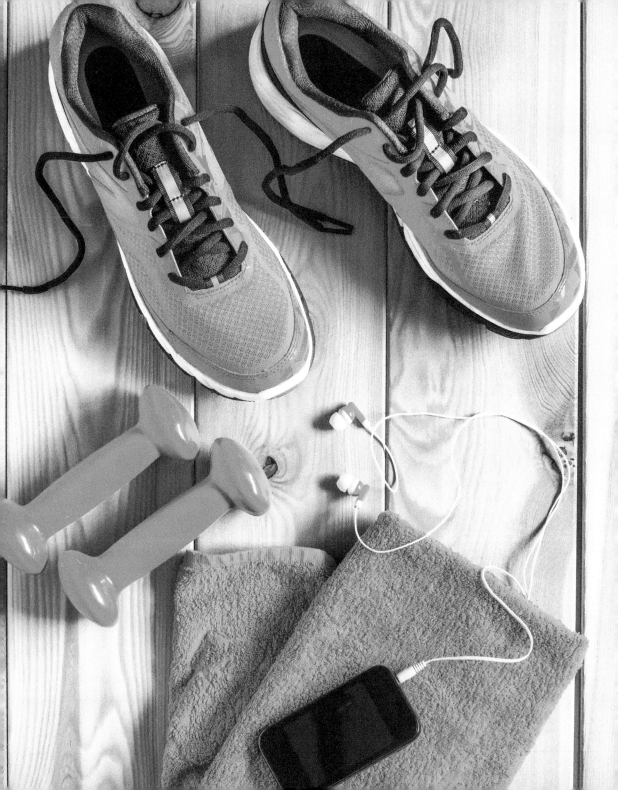

want you to be the great person you are; I just want you to be a slightly more active and health-conscious version.

No matter what weight I am (and I have been at different weights throughout my life), I would never want my goal to be a whole new me. I like me. The memory of being awkward and unfit informs my current fitness and health philosophy, fills me with empathy for everyone who is struggling to adopt a healthier lifestyle, and allows me to value my current, more confident self. Yes, if I stopped exercising, my goal would be to start again. But I wouldn't resolve to be a new person. My goal would be to still be me, but a version that was more consistent with her exercise routine.

Fifteen years after getting that YMCA membership I am still working through my health process. The only thing I know for sure is that there is no set end goal. No one gets to eventually win the health game and maintain his or her health while eating candy all day. Adopting and then maintaining a healthy lifestyle is a lifelong (and very rewarding) journey. I have had ebbs and flows of mindfulness and dedication. You will too. When you face an ebb, don't panic and don't give up. Persevere.

My clients and I joke that I am their personal cheerleader — I love cheering them on. I wish I could train every one

of you. But I can't, so I wrote this book. When you want to quit, pretend that I am in your living room saying, "You can do it!" Use the book in any way you find helpful. Read it from cover to cover to help you kick-start your health process, read a random chapter any time you need some extra pep in your step, or jump right to the "choose your own adventure" exercise program at the end of the book for a detailed plan of action. For extra motivation, stay connected to me through my website and newsletter or on Facebook, Twitter, and Pinterest. You will find all my contact information in the concluding chapter.

I KNOW you can be successful. Unfortunately, that is not enough. YOU need to know that you can be successful! Have you ever heard the joke "How many therapists does it take to change a light bulb? It takes one light bulb that wants to be changed"? Well, that joke applies to training as well. How many trainers does it take to change a light bulb? It takes one light bulb that not only wants to be changed, but that believes he or she can change and is willing to actively participate in that change.

You can evolve — you can adopt a healthier lifestyle — I know you can! Now, the question is, do you know you can? By the end of the book you will be thinking "Yes, Kathleen, I can!"

# My Philosophy

The fitness industry is profitable in large part because, to varying degrees, we all find it hard to motivate ourselves to make lifelong lifestyle changes. It doesn't matter if you're an avid exerciser or a newbie: finding the internal motivation to be active is hard.

Successfully adopting a healthier lifestyle is not about spending hours at the gym, finding the perfect diet, investing in every fad fitness product available, or judging yourself. The purpose of exercise should not be just to look fit. The goal of exercising should be to actually become fit. You will experience fewer aches and pains. It will increase your self-confidence. You will feel energized. Maybe you will gain the ability to play a sport you love, and you will be able to spend more quality active time with friends and family.

Some of you may have worked with a trainer before, but many of you probably have not. Not all trainers share my philosophy. Some yell, some focus only on working toward aesthetic goals, many think that more work is always better. I don't. I believe that more is not always better; I believe that better is better. My goal is to help you put together a workout routine that works best for you — your individual recipe for success.

Banish perfection from your vocabulary. The goal of being perfect — of following the perfect diet or working out every day — can be paralyzing. Plus, perfection is not possible; the goal of being perfect simply sets you up for failure. Instead, aim to be persistent, flexible, and patient.

Don't think that I am exempt from this reality. Yes, I love exercise, but *The Wire* and (gulp!) the original *Beverly Hills 90210* can still entice me to be lazy. I often have to use the motivational tricks found in chapter 2 to get through my workout. In the end, what makes me work out is that I know I will feel better if I move than if I don't.

Many of my clients tell me that although they are comfortable training with me, they don't want to go to their local gym on their own until they start to look fit. Many clients have even told me that they put off hiring a trainer because they did not feel fit enough. They were worried about being judged by the trainer.

Does this sound familiar? If so, the next time you're contemplating staying home because of what others will think, hear my voice saying, "Stop worrying about looking fit. It's not useful. Instead, care about becoming fit and energized. Fitness and health involve a lifelong learning process, not an end result. Don't let the fear of going to the gym sap your will to exercise."

Don't waste energy judging yourself or others. Instead, use that energy to get up and get moving. Open the door, step outside, and just move!

I too struggle with not judging myself. Once, when I was supposed to meet a friend for a boot camp class, I contemplated not going because I thought I was too tired to perform at my best. I actually emailed my friend and told her not to judge me during the class. How ridiculous and hypocritical. I almost allowed this self-judgment to keep me from working out, but I didn't. Instead, I told myself that I would feel better if I moved. And I did. I always do. I live by the rule that the worse your mood, the more important your workout.

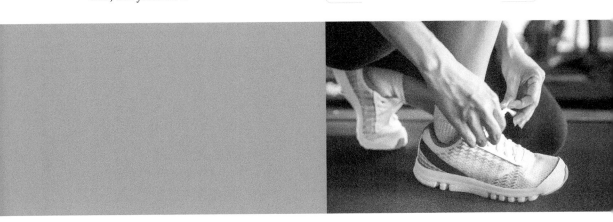

# What You Can Expect In This Book

. . . . . . . . . . . . . . . . . . . . . . . . . . . . . . . . . . . . . . . . . . . . . . . . . .

I can't tell you how excited I am to share my fifteen years of health knowledge and experience with you!

My hope is that my book will convey my health philosophy, teach you accessible fitness knowledge, provide you with tools you can use to motivate yourself to move more, and give you a practical health plan you can use to jump-start your new, healthier lifestyle. I suggest you use my advice to create a month-long plan, versus a two-week plan. I personally like making thirty-day goals. The time frame is long enough for you to start seeing positive results but short enough that it doesn't seem overwhelming.

In the first ten chapters, I offer information and motivational tricks that will help you put together your unique recipe for health success. In the final chapter of the book, I help you form your unique plan of action — your recipe for health success. As you read, imagine that I'm in your living room training you and encouraging you to get fit while still having fun. Throughout the book I include "Kathleenisms." A Kathleenism is a succinct way of describing a given element of my philosophy. My goal is for my clients — and now for you — to remember the Kathleenisms and use them as inspiration to make healthier

choices on a daily basis. When you read the Kathleenisms, imagine that I am beside you encouraging you to persevere.

In chapter 1, "How to Set Yourself Up for Health Success," I discuss why you have to actively set yourself up for health success, and how to actually do it. The key word is actively. Adopting a healthier lifestyle isn't a passive process. Among other things, I suggest scheduling your workouts in advance and trying to anticipate and troubleshoot potential setbacks. If you don't take the time to set yourself up for success, you might as well be setting yourself up for failure.

Improved health often feels like an uphill battle at the best of times. You don't need to be your own roadblock.

In chapter 2, "Make Daily Movement Non-Negotiable," I explain how to change your mindset about activity so that daily movement becomes non-negotiable. Instead of thinking of movement as an if, I teach you how to frame moving as a when.

Chapter 3 is titled "Some Movement Is Always Better Than No Movement." The main take-away is that since there will never be the perfect week to start exercising, start looking for daily opportunities to be active. Every bit of motion adds up, and every situation can be reframed as an opportunity for movement. The following four strategies will help you weave movement into your life: the "piggyback" strategy, tracking steps, doing "posture-friendly" exercises throughout the day, and taking the colour challenge.

Chapter 4, "Make Fitness Goals, Not Fitness Wishes," points to the fact that for most of us it's easier to talk about our health and fitness goals than to actually make them a reality. Who hasn't uttered unrealistic statements regarding their health, such as "Come Monday, no more junk food"? I know I have. These types of bold statements are examples of what I call fitness wishes. Wishes are akin to hoping a genie will magically make you healthier.

Don't get me wrong — wishes can be a great first step, but without a concrete implementation plan, wishes will most likely be forgotten as soon as life takes over. And life always takes over. The trick to making your fitness wishes a reality is to establish realistic goals. In chapter 4 I teach you how to do exactly that.

Chapter 5 is titled "Adopting a Healthier Lifestyle Is a Marathon, Not a Sprint." Too many of us buy into the myth that you can lose weight quickly and then keep it off easily. This sets us up for health failure. Unhealthy habits are not formed in a day. It is unrealistic to think they can be replaced overnight.

To change your lifestyle for good, you need to "buy in" for the long haul. To do this, you have to learn how to change your

I always tell my clients, "When you fall off the 'fitness horse,' don't give up. Use it as a learning experience and get back on a more informed rider."

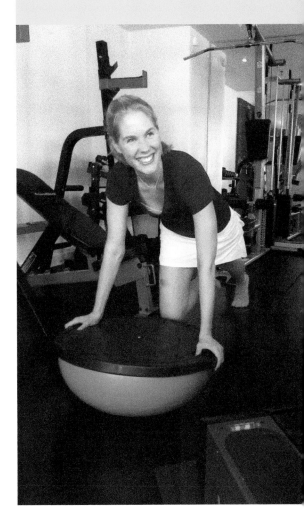

attitude toward exercise. Recalibrate your expectations. Understand that you are actively choosing to make healthier choices; you are not being forced to eat vegetables. In fact, being able to eat healthier food is a privilege. "Embrace the marathon," and recognize that to survive a marathon, you need to change your attitude toward health.

Instead of trying to find the miracle fix, aim to have a greater number of healthy habits this month than you had last month so that you slowly find a new, healthier normal. In chapter 6, "Find the WWHH of Your Eating Habits and Adopt the Captain Obvious Approach to Health," I state the truth that no one wants to hear: Adopting a healthier lifestyle is not as simple as finding the perfect diet to follow and/or being disciplined. I wish it were, but it isn't, and anyone who tells you that probably wants to sell you something. Our eating habits are tied to our emotions, our established habits, our lifestyle, and our childhood eating habits. Maintaining a healthier lifestyle long term involves figuring out the WWHH of your eating habits — WHAT you eat, WHY you eat, HOW you eat, and HOW MUCH you eat. The operative word is you.

You can stress eat or binge eat out of loneliness on any diet — lots of people overeat gluten-free cake and Paleo treats. If you don't become aware of your eating patterns, your personal food habits will simply follow you from nutrition program to nutrition program. In chapter 6 I outline the steps needed to explore your unique relationship with food so that you can tailor a healthy lifestyle plan that is sustainable for and unique to you.

In chapter 7, "Establish a Health Entourage," I detail the usefulness of having what I call a "health entourage," and how to go about setting one up. A health entourage is a personalized network of support; it can include supportive friends and family, a fitness buddy, an accountability buddy, a nutrition buddy, or even an entire fitness club. Everyone needs to find ways to set themselves up for health and fitness success. A health entourage helps you do just that.

Chapter 8 is titled "Stop Fixating on the Scale and Aim to Get Out of Body Debt." The main take-away is to stop fixating on reaching a certain weight and/or conflating thinness with health. Fixating on the weight on the scale — and using "health" interchangeably with "thinness" — is ultimately not healthy or helpful. The scale doesn't differentiate water or muscle loss from fat loss, and losing weight in an unhealthy way — even when weight loss is needed — is not beneficial to your long-term physical or psychological health.

Make your health goal to get out of "body debt" by amassing "body credit." Body credit is each individual's level of energy, vitality, and physical resilience.

You accumulate credit by making healthy choices. You deplete your credit by consciously or unconsciously making unhealthy choices, such as sitting for hours, going on extreme diets, or eating unhealthfully. Body debt occurs when your unhealthy habits outnumber your healthy habits. You are in debt if you consistently feel like you are moving through mud, if you injure easily and recovery slowly, if you almost always feel cranky, if you can't sleep, and if you have a hard time maintaining or losing weight. Losing weight on the scale may be one part of decreasing your debt, but your weight is only one small part of the debt-credit system of health. Focus on getting out of debt by making as many healthy choices as possible — sleep more, eat nutritionally dense foods, move more, and sit less. Aim to feel strong, powerful, and energized.

I call chapter 9 "Ways You Might Be Unknowingly Sabotaging Your Progress." It is one thing not to reach your goals if you are eating fries every day and skipping workouts, but it is extremely frustrating to work hard and still not succeed. In chapter 9 I outline four reasons why you might not be seeing results despite your best efforts. The four reasons are not doing strength training, getting inadequate recovery, ignoring the importance of high-intensity interval workouts, and a lack of mindfulness.

It just plain sucks to give it your all and still not reach your health goals. If you feel like you are always diligent but never successful, this chapter is for you.

In chapter 10, "Variety Is the Spice of Life," I explain how to stay motivated and avoid the dreaded fitness plateau. Many people stop training out of boredom, but working out can and SHOULD be fun (or at least not tedious). Of course you're going to quit if you find exercise boring — disliking something is a huge disincentive. My mission in chapter 10 is to describe a variety of different workouts in the hope that a few will intrigue you. I want you to discover one or two workouts that you like (or at least one you don't hate) so that you are inspired to work out for the rest of your life.

Chapter 11 is my grand finale — the pièce de résistance. In it I connect all the dots. I give you the practical guidelines you need to create and then implement your individual health recipe. I call chapter 11 "The 'Choose Your Own Adventure' Exercise Program." No cookie-cutter plans here! First you decide what "exercise personality" you are: a gym bunny, a competitive athletic gym bunny, a time-crunched multi-tasker, or a homebody. Then you build your unique routine — a program built around your reality, rhythms, lifestyle, and personal goals. This chapter offers you the benefits of both structure and flexibility; you build a practical, structured program that melds with your distinctive lifestyle and personality quirks.

# CHAPTER TAKE-AWAY

Adopting a healthier lifestyle is not just about making one change, such as eating chia seeds, cutting out gluten, or doing crunches. Think big picture. You need to sit less, become more mindful of your daily health habits, improve your nutrition, and move more.

The trick to successfully adopting a healthier lifestyle long term is creating a recipe for success that is tailored to your individual body and your lifestyle; always remember that your age, gender, activity level, nutritional habits, genetics, and fitness and health history will affect how you respond to exercise.

Learn to appreciate and love your body. Appreciate your genetic window. Work to be the best possible version of yourself. Become fit because you want to become healthier, not simply out of a desire to look like your favourite actress or model. Regardless of how your appearance changes because of exercise, moving will make you feel better.

By this point, I hope you're feeling motivated, and possibly slightly excited, to get moving. More important, I hope you're feeling that becoming more active is within the realm of possibility. Adopting a healthier lifestyle is possible and you can be successful. Don't let negative self-talk derail your progress. If you're feeling overwhelmed, tell yourself that the first step is to simply read this book. Don't get ahead of yourself. You don't have to change all of your health habits immediately. Remind yourself that just reading this introduction is a positive step forward. Adopting a healthier lifestyle is all about moving in the right direction, about "trending positive." Now get up, take a walk around your living room, and come back to read some more!

# CHAPTER I

# HOW TO SET YOURSELF UP FOR HEALTH SUCCESS

Adopting a healthier lifestyle isn't a passive process. Improved health doesn't just happen.

At least once per week someone tells me they wish they had my discipline, as if discipline was something I was lucky enough to have been born with or to have found on the side of the road. Believe me, I wasn't born disciplined. I have actively learned how to be someone who (mostly) puts my health first.

Note that I used the word actively. Adopting a healthier lifestyle doesn't just happen; you have to be actively involved in creating the healthier version of yourself that you want to be. You have to actively set yourself up for health success.

I used to actively make unhealthy choices. Now, I not only consciously make healthier choices, I actually plan my life so that healthy choices are the easier choices.

You, like me, can adopt a healthier lifestyle. I KNOW you can. By reading this book, you are already trending positive. Next, embrace the reality that improved health doesn't just happen; you have to make it happen.

## Kathleen's Seven Strategies to Set Yourself Up for Health Success (abbreviated version)

**1.** Stop aspiring to health and training perfection. Perfection is not possible.

**2.** Remember the two Cs: Make your workouts convenient so that you do them consistently.

**3.** Work toward finding your exercise "bliss"; find things that you like to do so that training no longer feels like an obligation.

**4.** Figure out your WHY. Find your "health dream" — the emotional reason why you want to move.

**5.** Flip your negative thoughts; turn "I don't want to train" into "I am so lucky that I get to train."

**6.** Find your inner athlete; learn to be proud of what your body can do, not just of how it looks.

**7.** Mindfulness + Preparation = Success. Become mindful of your particular health pitfalls so that you can prepare solutions in advance.

# Kathleen's Seven Strategies to Set Yourself Up for Health Success (detailed version)

. . . . . . . . . . . . . . . . . . . . . . . . . . . . . . . . . . . . . . . . . . .

## Strategy 1 — Stop aspiring to perfection

Aiming for perfection simply sets you up for failure — perfection is not possible.

Since there is no way to be perfect, we often do one of two things. We let ourselves either consciously or unconsciously off the hook before we even start, by thinking that we will fail, so why try? Or we aim for perfection, then when we can't live up to our unrealistic goals, we fall back into our negative health habits. The goal of "perfect" is like giving yourself a built-in excuse to throw in the "workout towel" when something doesn't go according to plan.

Either way, the main take-away is that you need to stop trying to find the perfect week to start exercising or the perfect time to work out, or assuming that every workout has to unfold according to plan. Stop saying things like, "This week is already too full; there is no point trying to start working out. I will train next week." You can always find time to walk for ten minutes. Remember my favourite Kathleenism: Some movement is always better than no movement. Ten minutes of walking is better than nothing. Skipping a workout often kick-starts a negative domino effect; one week of inactivity turns into a month of inactivity, and before you know it, an entire season has gone by. You feel in worse shape

An "all or nothing" or "perfection or nothing" approach to health too often leads to binge eating and unhappiness. Think about adopting the 80/20 rule of healthy living. Tell yourself that as long as you are good 80 percent of the time, you can still enjoy less-healthy options 20 percent of the time. Be as healthy as you can, as often as you can, but allow yourself to be human. As I tell my clients, perfection is what you expect from machines, and, thankfully, we are not robots.

and heavier than ever, which means it is even harder to start training again.

If you can't make your spin class or do your entire gym routine, don't abandon ship altogether. Stop thinking that every workout has to go exactly according to plan to be worthwhile. Go for a walk or a mini-run, or do a few exercises at home. Just do something. Consistency beats perfection.

Don't misunderstand me. I am not arguing that you shouldn't have goals. Abandoning the quest for perfection is not about abandoning goal setting. I am a firm believer in making realistic, sustainable goals. I will discuss goal setting in detail in chapter 4, but in short, part of staying on a positive health track is having realistic goals while also being flexible. Modify your plans as life dictates, and when you fall off the fitness wagon — it is bound to happen once or twice — assess why and then get right back on track. Such a large component of being happy and successful in life is setting realistic expectations. So, instead of being surprised and discouraged by setbacks, expect them. Then make sure you learn from them. Reframe the experience: You didn't fail, you had a great learning experience. Note what went wrong and then aim to actively make smarter goals and choices next time. Play around; figure out what type of goal setting, motivational strategies, support networks, and scheduling strategies work for you.

Remind yourself that people who successfully make long-term lifestyle changes aren't usually successful the first time. They don't succeed by being perfect, they succeed because they persevere. Health is a process — a non-linear one at that. It takes daily dedication.

Basically, ditch the goal of perfection. Instead, aim to be persistent, flexible, and patient.

## Strategy 2 Remember the two Cs of training: convenience and consistency

Make your workouts convenient so that you do them consistently. One fantastic way to make your workout convenient is to set up a home gym.

I often get asked, "What workout is best?" My answer is not flashy or exciting.

The best workout is the one you can do consistently. Convenience, not fancy, expensive equipment, is key. A workout can be touted as the most intense and "best" workout, but if you can't (or won't) do it consistently, it is not actually the best workout for you. To achieve any health and fitness goal you need to be consistently active.

The more convenient the workout, the more likely you are to stick with it.

So pick an activity that is convenient — don't forget to consider location, timing, and duration. The yoga studio around the corner might be conveniently located, but if you never make a class because they are too lengthy to be convenient, the benefits are moot.

So how do you make activity more convenient? First, stop thinking that exercise has to take place in a gym to be worthwhile. Any time you are moving, you are not sitting — sitting negatively affects your health. When it comes to movement, remember that something is always better than nothing. Find ways to make movement (of any duration) convenient so that you will move consistently. Let's take the example of the inconvenient yoga classes. Instead of giving up on yoga altogether, a good compromise might be to download a yoga podcast or get a DVD to do at home.

One way to make exercise convenient is to set up a home gym. Sure, an actual gym will always have fancier machines, but if you never actually get to the gym to use them, the quality of the equipment is irrelevant. Even with minimal equipment, a home gym is a great way to set yourself up for success. It ensures that you can always do something because it decreases the structural obstacles that keep you from working out. When you don't have time to waste getting to and from the gym, do a workout at home.

If you love the idea of going to an actual gym, great; get a membership. Go when you can, but when life takes over, to stay consistent, train at home. The key thing to remember is that moving is non-negotiable; do whatever it takes to fit movement into your schedule.

You can put together a decent gym without spending a ton of money. Get your cardio in by running or walking outside. Or run up and down the stairs in your building. Or buy a mini-trampoline. They are fun, low impact, don't take up a huge amount of room, are fairly inexpensive, and are a great complement to running or walking outside.

You can do a full-body strength workout by using your own body as resistance. Take a look at chapter 11 for a detailed program; you will find the workout in the "homebody" exercise program.

If you are worried that you will get bored doing only body-weight exercises, invest in one or more of the following pieces:

**A RESISTANCE BAND** Light, inexpensive, portable, and have almost limitless possibilities.

**A STABILITY BALL** Put your head and shoulders on it while you do dumbbell bench presses, or do push-ups and crunches on it.

**FREE WEIGHTS** Start with light weights and buy heavier ones as you get stronger.

**FOAM ROLLER** A long cylindrical object made of foam. Fantastic for anyone who sits at a desk.

**A SITFIT** An inflatable cushion that looks somewhat like a Whoopee cushion.

## Sample Resistance-Band Exercise

**STANDING ROWS:**
➡ Loop the band around a stationary object. Hold one end of the band in each hand. Use your upper back to row your elbows backward until your wrists touch either side of your chest. Slowly release.

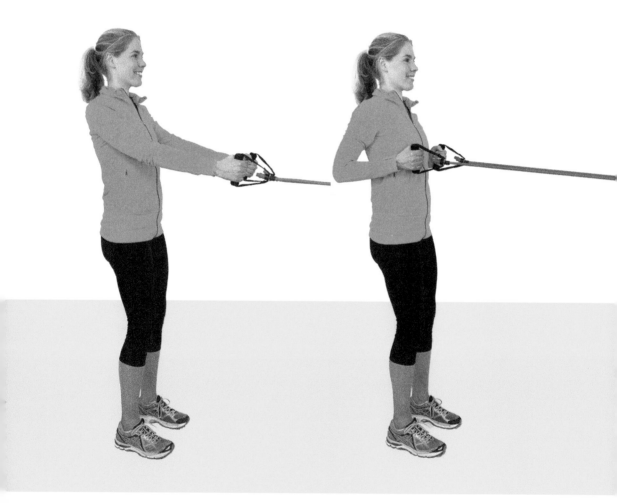

## Sample Stability-Ball and Free-Weight Exercise

**STABILITY-BALL BENCH PRESS:**

➡ Put your head and shoulders on the ball, feet on the floor. Lift your hips up and engage your bum. Your lower back should be in a neutral position, core engaged. Don't push through your lower back — push through your bum.

➡ Hold one dumbbell in each hand, arms straight and directly above your chest. Slowly lower the weights until your elbows are at ninety degrees while keeping your hips up. If you don't have dumbbells, use soup cans or water bottles.

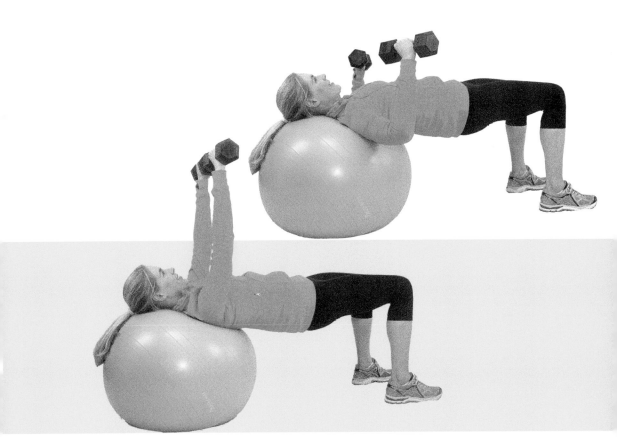

## Sample Foam-Roller Exercise

**CHEST STRETCH:**

⮕ Lie on the roller lengthwise with your head at one end and your bum at the other, and
spread your arms out to the side. Hold the stretch for thirty seconds.

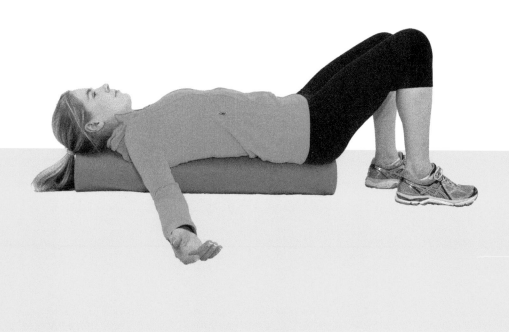

## Sample SitFit Exercise

➡ Sit on it at your desk to help correct posture imbalances. Put it on your desk chair and try to keep the SitFit's air evenly distributed as you sit.

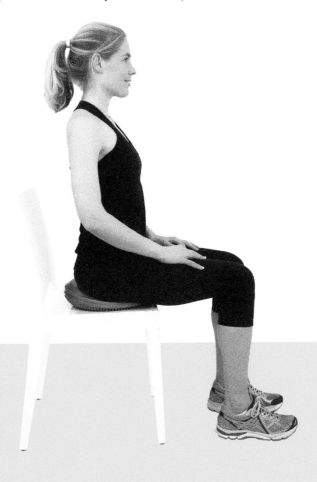

If setting up a home gym isn't for you, no problem. Download a yoga or Pilates podcast or pick up a DVD, go for a walk with your dogs, play a sport with your kids, or simply walk to work. Figure out a way to make your workout convenient so that you will do it consistently. Just do something — anything!

# Strategy 3 Work toward finding your exercise bliss

Find your exercise "bliss." Your bliss is something that you actually WANT to do, something you don't want to miss. If you like your workout, you are more likely to stick with it over the long term and incorporate it into the fabric of your life.

Understanding workouts as an obligation or as drudgery just sets us up for failure. You are way more likely to search for reasons to "skip" if you hate the workout. Plus, I know that when I feel like I have to do something — when it feels like a chore — I am more likely to have a reaction akin to adolescent rebellion. I resist (usually unconsciously) because I don't like being told how I should live my life.

Now, finding your bliss doesn't mean you will always jump at being active. There are some days I don't want to run — and I LOVE running. On those days,

Ways to make exercise enjoyable

- If you like friendly competition, join a sports team.
- If you know you like a particular type of class — like yoga or Zumba — make fitness dates with friends.
- If you love your dog, structure a workout around your daily dog walks.
- If you get pleasure from watching your kids accomplishing something, practise their sport with them. Both of you benefit. Win-win!
- Structure family fun time around being active. In the summer, go for bike rides or hikes. In the winter, try skiing or skating.
- Dance around in your living room.
- Learn a new skill such as line dancing or ballet.
- Make active dates with your partner or spouse.

try the motivation strategies I teach you in chapter 2. They will put some extra pep in your step.

# Strategy 4 Figure out your WHY

Figure out what your health dream is — the emotional reason why you want to be more active. Write your dream down. Read it when you need some extra motivation.

I am not talking about why your doctor or partner thinks you should be active. Those are their reasons, not yours. Plus, expert-inspired reasons, such as those from your doctor, tend to be very intellectualized. It is easy to find intellectual and rational reasons why you should exercise. We all know that exercise and eating well are good for our health. In my experience, those reasons will motivate most people to be good when they aren't hungry, tired, stressed, or angry. When life takes over and emotions are high, most of us need more than an intellectual reason to stay on track.

Find a strong personal, emotional reason you want to move — your WHY. That way, when life takes over, you can remind yourself of the WHY and you will be more likely to make healthy choices.

## Possible WHY goals

- To strength train so that you will be strong enough to play with your grandkids.
- To strength train to improve your performance in your sport.
- To improve your balance so that you don't fall on the ice and potentially break something.
- To train so that you can go on an active vacation with your spouse.
- To decrease pain.

Every night, make a list of the positive choices you made that day that brought you closer to achieving your WHY goal. Brainstorm how you can replicate your positive choices. List the choices you made that were not ideal and figure out how you can avoid them in future. See chapter 5 for more information regarding the importance of finding and focusing on positive health choices.

My dream is to run injury-free for life. Picturing myself running at ninety helps motivate me to lift weights, eat well, stretch, and get enough sleep. I find having a health dream — a WHY — extremely motivating. Try it. It can't hurt!

## Strategy 5 Flip your negative thoughts

Flip your negative thoughts! Be strict with yourself — make yourself turn "I don't want to train" into "I am so lucky that I get to train."

Hopefully, after reading strategies 3 and 4, you have already come up with a few activities that you actually enjoy and have started to brainstorm your WHY. Unfortunately, even armed with both these strategies you are still going to have days when you just don't want to train; we all do. Even I sometimes think, "I don't want to train. I want to watch TV."

When I don't feel like training I flip my thoughts. I tell myself, "Kathleen, stop being a negative Nelly. Exercise is not something you have to do; it is something you GET to do! Moving is a privilege. You are so lucky that you get to go for a run today!"

Basically, I talk myself into feeling grateful for the fact that I have the ability to move. If I really need an extra push, I remind myself how much I hated not being able to run while recovering from a minor hip injury two years ago. I wanted to run, but I couldn't. I craved moving when I couldn't move.

So, the next time you don't want to exercise, try to flip it. Lecture yourself. Reframe how you understand working out — think about being active as something you "get to do" versus something you "have to do." A large part of adopting a healthier lifestyle is modifying one's attitude toward exercise, and flipping it helps you do just that. If flipping it doesn't work for you, don't worry, chapter 5 is filled with other ways you can change your attitude toward moving. One of these strategies will work for you.

## Strategy 6 Find your inner athlete

I am not suggesting that to successfully adopt a healthier lifestyle you have to push your body to the limits in the way most serious athletes do. I am not even arguing that you have to start playing a sport. Your sport might be walking. What I am saying is, athletes have found a way to thrive on being active. So learn from them; steal their strategies.

## Find your inner athlete

- Identify as someone who is active. Most athletes identify as someone who is active; they gain confidence and self-worth from being strong and healthy. I am active in large part because I see myself, and I know that others see me, as someone who is fit and strong. The pride and the self-worth I gain from being active motivate me to continue.
- Lesson for the non-athlete: Start to think of yourself as someone who is active. When you contemplate skipping a workout, ask yourself, "Am I the type of person who skips, or am I the type of person who works out?" Most of my long-term clients who have successfully adopted a healthier lifestyle continue to be active in part because they identify as someone who is active. They have, in one way or another, found their "inner athlete." Find yours.
- Take an off-season. Athletes take an off-season to recharge physically and emotionally. They don't sit on the sofa; they use their off-season to recover, do unstructured training, cross-train, and work on any physical weak links.
- Lesson for the non-athlete: Repeating the same routine over and over can be draining physically and mentally. So switch things up. If you always go to spin classes, try a Zumba class. If you always run, try lifting weights.
- Strength train. Athletes know that strength training helps maintain joint integrity, limit injury, improve athletic performance, and increase muscle mass.
- Lesson for the non-athlete: Don't do just cardio. Strength train.
- Establish short- and long-term goals so that your workouts have a purpose. Athletes have short- and long-term goals. In order to achieve their goals, they develop a training plan. Every workout has a purpose. Even "easy" days have a purpose — they allow the athlete to recharge physically and mentally. I find having a specific purpose attached to each workout ensures that I am invested in the workout, which makes me less likely to skip training.

- Lesson for the non-athlete: Develop goals and a workout plan. Following a program will help you stay motivated and allow you to track your progress. I discuss goal setting in more detail in chapter 4. In chapter 11 I outline how to develop a personalized workout plan.
- Athletes establish physical, performance-based goals, not just aesthetic goals. Athletes know that to be successful at their sport they have to make performance-related goals. Their goals are not simply connected to how their body looks.
- Lesson for the non-athlete: Purely aesthetic goals can negatively impact a person's self-confidence and body image. Plus, when someone makes only aesthetic goals, they often inadequately fuel their body and ultimately don't stay active over the long term. Sure, have an aesthetic goal if that matters to you, but also make performance-related goals. Aim to be able to do a certain number of push-ups or to strengthen your core.

## Strategy 7 Mindfulness + Preparation = Success

Adopting a healthy lifestyle is not about "discipline"; it is about mindfulness and preparation. Meaning, become mindful of YOUR particular health pitfalls so that you can prepare solutions in advance. Once you have identified your individual triggers, tailor an individualized game plan. When it comes to exercise, take as many steps as possible to set yourself up for fitness success. In terms of diet, become aware of what I call the WWHH of your diet: WHAT, WHY, HOW, and HOW MUCH you eat — and then figure out appropriate measures. For example, I make bad choices — and get really crabby — when I let myself get too hungry. So I always carry a healthy snack to make sure I don't grab the closest chocolate bar. For a more detailed explanation of the WWHH of healthy eating, see chapter 6.

## If you do this ____, your solution is ____.

**If you have a particular food trigger (for me it is chocolate):**

Don't keep your food trigger at home or at work.

**If you make bad choices when you travel:**

Pack a travel blender and protein powder. Since most hotels have ice, and bananas are usually accessible, you can always make a protein shake if needed.

Go grocery shopping as soon as you arrive at your destination. Buy healthy snacks for your hotel room.

On road trips, don't let yourself fall into the trap of "having to" buy unhealthy snacks. Research healthier restaurants that are en route or, better yet, pack a cooler full of nutritious snacks.

**If you make bad choices when you go to restaurants:**

Look at the menu online and decide what you will have before you get there. When you arrive, don't even open the menu; just order whatever you have already decided on.

**If you tend to snack when bored:**

Don't keep food on your office desk or on your kitchen counter. If food is within sight or is convenient, you are more likely to grab it.

**If you know that you are a social eater:**

Stay hydrated. Sip water all through your cocktail party. That way you won't mistake dehydration for hunger.

If you are attending an event at someone's home, offer to bring something. That way, you'll have at least one healthy option.

**If you tend to slack off while on vacation:**

Research interesting local sites in advance that you can explore on foot or on a bike. Use the pedometer on your phone or buy a tracking device and aim to get 10,000 steps per day.

Pack workout clothes and a resistance band so that you don't even have to find a gym. Train in your hotel room.

It is always possible to make healthier choices; it just takes mindfulness and some advance planning. On Sundays look at your week, identify possibly situations where you might fall off the fitness horse, and then form a plan of action. If you make a choice you are not proud of, use it as a learning experience. Make a more informed choice next time, and remember, one indulgence doesn't have to turn into a night or day full of indulgences.

# CHAPTER TAKE-AWAY

Don't try to implement all these strategies at once — that would be too overwhelming. Pick one or two and start there. Try implementing the two Cs of training (convenience and consistency); for example, walk home from the subway every day. Once that strategy is your "normal," add another one.

Remember, your negative health habits were not formed in a day. You will not form healthier habits overnight. If you catch yourself thinking, "Where on earth do I start?" tell yourself to just START! Get up and pace the room, walk around the block, dance. Do something — anything! When it comes to movement, remember: Some movement is always better than no movement.

# CHAPTER 2

# MAKE DAILY MOVEMENT NON-NEGOTIABLE

The worse your mood,
the more important your workout.

"The worse your mood, the more important your workout" is probably the Kathleenism that I personally find the most useful. I use it daily; I repeat it to myself like a mantra whenever I'm contemplating skipping my workout. My other mantra is "You are not the type of person who picks watching TV over exercising. If you want to watch a show, either watch it after your workout, or get on your bike and watch it as you cycle." The main take-away of both mantras is that movement is non-negotiable.

I define non-negotiables as life events that, for the most part, you just do. You don't seriously contemplate if you should or shouldn't do them; they seem natural — a part of your everyday.

Everyone's non-negotiables differ slightly. Some people decide that saving a set amount of money each month is non-negotiable. Others decide that a daily family dinner is a must. Most people don't question if they should go to work or pick their children up from school. One is not born understanding these events as non-negotiable, but they become an unquestioned part of our identity and routine.

Moving and eating well are two of my personal non-negotiables, but they have not always been. Even now, after years of learning to love exercise, I still don't always jump for joy before a workout. I do, however, know that I will ALWAYS feel better after working out — which is largely why I am no longer as tempted to skip as I once was. I used to do maybe 75 percent of my scheduled workouts. Now I do maybe 97 percent. I'm proud of that percentage, but it took work. My follow-through rate increased because I gradually changed the structure of my life and, possibly more important, I shifted my mindset so that daily movement became one of my non-negotiables. It became a non-negotiable partly because I can honestly tell myself that I will be a happier, peppier version of Kathleen when I move — and the more of a funk I am in, the more of a non-negotiable I know my workout is.

My body has a kinesthetic memory of how great I feel post-workout. Years of experience have taught me not only to push through the "will I or won't I" phase of my internal exercise question, but also to try not to even allow the question to enter my head. This relates to a point I have already made — that maintaining a healthier lifestyle takes perseverance, and that it is not simply enough to work through challenging times, you also have to learn from your mistakes. A Kathleenism you'll see me repeat many times throughout this book is, when you fall off the fitness horse, don't give up. Use it as a learning experience and get back on a more informed rider. Setbacks are inevitable. You can either be discouraged by them and let them defeat you, or you can learn from them. The former is not helpful; the latter is. Learn from setbacks: use your experiences as building blocks in your quest to make healthy eating and movement non-negotiable.

To do this, we have to change the way you frame the exercise debate in your head. Notice that I said "we" — I'm invested in your fitness mission too. I want everyone to succeed and feel more energized and empowered. My ultimate goal is to minimize the times you have the internal "will I or won't I exercise today" debate. To do this, we have to reframe the "exercise question" in your head.

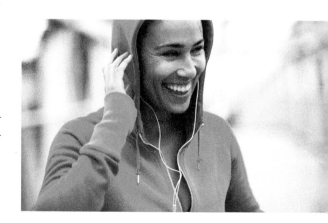

Stop saying, "Will I exercise today?" Instead say, "WHEN will I exercise today?"

Tell yourself, "I AM the type of person who makes working out a priority!"

Substituting when for if may seem like a silly semantic change, but it's not! Asking yourself, "Will I exercise today?" gives you a loophole, an option to skip moving altogether. People who ask themselves, "Will I exercise?" give themselves the okay to decide that today is not the day to move. Let's look at the following scenario: You sleep past your alarm and miss your workout, so you think, "Crap, too bad. I have plans after work, so I guess I can't work out today." That's the thought process of someone who asks themselves, "Will I exercise?"

Now, imagine this scenario instead: You sleep past your alarm. You wake up and say to yourself, "That's too bad, but since not moving is not an option, what is my plan B? When will I exercise?" In the second scenario, the person fits in movement by going for a walk at lunch, taking the stairs throughout the day, and doing core work on the floor in the evening as their kids play. Sure, they didn't get to do their full workout and, yes, a full workout may have been ideal, but aiming for perfection is not usually useful. The fact that a full workout would have been better is a moot point because it didn't happen. In scenario two, at least the person didn't give up. They formed a contingency plan and did something. Not moving was simply not an option. The next step in their fitness journey is to analyze if their original goal of training in the morning is realistic. If training in the morning is an unrealistic goal, they will continue to miss workouts, so they might need to rethink that goal. I discuss goal setting in detail in chapter 4. Get excited!

Challenge yourself to move every day for a month, even if you just walk home from work. After thirty days, moving will have become a habit, you will have found ways that exercise can easily fit into your life, and you will know how good it makes you feel.

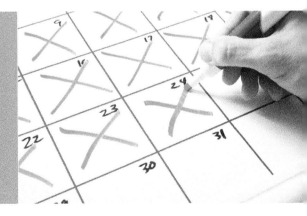

Thinking, "When will I exercise today?" makes movement non-negotiable.

Now, I get it — if you've never worked out, the idea of daily non-negotiable movement is probably daunting. It can be hard to make yourself move when you're not in the habit of exercising. I remember how hard it was at the beginning. My mom had to drag me to the gym. The good news is that it does become easier. Once you have established a habit, you're less likely to ask yourself that "will I or won't I" question. Plus, when you exercise regularly you develop a kinesthetic memory of how great you feel post-workout, which will help motivate you to exercise.

I've been able to make movement non-negotiable because for the past fifteen years or so I've learned from my health mistakes and gotten right back on the horse. Through some successes and many errors I've learned what works for me. I've consciously formed positive habits that create an environment where daily movement and healthy eating can both be non-negotiable. The three key words from the above sentence are learned, consciously, and habits. Apply the information I suggest in chapter 1 to learn how to consciously create healthy habits and how to set yourself up for success. Once you're set up for success, understanding daily movement as non-negotiable will be that much easier.

Set yourself up for success. Take the time to establish an environment where movement and healthy eating become a "when," not an "if." For example, I make exercise dates with friends so that exercising is fun. I sign up for races so that I am both monetarily and emotionally invested in exercise. I always keep things like cut-up vegetables, fruit, cooked chicken, and beans in my kitchen so that I can easily whip up a healthy meal, and most important, I NEVER bring unhealthy food home. I know that if I am exhausted after a long run, I am more likely to mindlessly overindulge on whatever is in my fridge. So I don't give myself that option. I simply don't keep things like chocolate–peanut butter ice cream in the house.

# How Can You Make Movement and Healthier Eating Non-Negotiable?

First, try to implement the concrete steps I outlined in chapter 1. To review:

1. Stop aiming for health and training perfection. Perfection is not possible.

2. Remember the two Cs. Make your workouts convenient so that you do them consistently.

3. Work toward finding your exercise bliss; find things that you LIKE to do so that training no longer feels like an obligation.

4. Find your health dream — the emotional reason WHY you want to move.

5. Flip your negative thoughts; turn "I don't want to train" into "I am so lucky that I get to train."

6. Find your inner athlete; learn to be proud of what your body can do, not just of how it looks.

7. Mindfulness + Preparation = Success. Become mindful of your particular health pitfalls so that you can prepare solutions in advance.

These steps are described in more detail in chapter 1. Following them will help you create healthier habits and thus an environment where daily movement can become one of your non-negotiables. Soon you will think of moving like brushing your teeth — something you don't even contemplate not doing; you just do it!

Now, as I stated earlier, I have not always considered moving and eating well non-negotiables. I have spent fifteen years making them my non-negotiables. Even now it sometimes takes more than these seven tips to keep me on track. Whenever I feel like I am slipping backward in my health journey, or I am frustrated with my progress, I remember these next four tips. They help me continue to make movement and healthy eating non-negotiable, even when I just want to sit on the sofa and eat chocolate.

Never give up on making moving and eating well non-negotiable!

# Tips on How to Persevere

. . . . . . . . . . . . . . . . . . . . . . . . . . . . . . . . . . . . . . . . . . . . . . . . . . . . . . . . . .

1. Aim to trend positive. Instead of falling into the all-too-common trap of making unrealistic health goals, simply aim to trend positive. Aim to make more healthy choices this month than you did last month. If you miss a workout, don't worry. Instead of feeling frustrated, learn from your mistake. Don't let yourself get frustrated; perfection is not possible. Instead, decide not to miss two workouts. Get right back on the fitness horse and aim to miss fewer workouts this month than you did last month.

2. Stay in your own lane. Your health process is exactly that — YOUR health process. Don't get caught up in what trendy diets your friends are trying or not trying. When you go out to eat with friends or family, don't let their choices dictate your choices. Plan in advance what you will drink and eat, then don't give in to peer pressure. Don't be judgmental of your friends when they want to eat and drink, but don't eat cake in solidarity with them. Be your own health boss — stay in your own lane.

3. When you want to indulge, use my "love it" rule. Go ahead, treat yourself — life is worth living, and deprivation often leads to binge eating — but before you do, ask yourself two questions: "Do I love it?" and "Is this an appropriate portion?" Have an appropriate portion of something you love, not just of whatever is around. Don't gorge; you can always have another moderate portion tomorrow. Treat yourself to things you LOVE, and indulge in moderation. Don't feel guilty; enjoy your treat.

4. Prioritize getting enough sleep. The less you sleep, the more ghrelin hormone your body produces, which means that your appetite will increase. Plus, you will produce less leptin, which is the hormone that helps your body feel satiated. Getting adequate amounts of sleep can help control your weight and will make it easier for healthier eating to become a non-negotiable. Often, when I feel my health resolve slipping, it is because I am tired. If it is late at night and I want sugar, I try to instead just go to sleep. I always wake up the next day with a new resolve to make movement and healthy eating non-negotiable.

A few years ago I recorded my mood before and after workouts for two weeks. Each time, I recorded a higher number after my workout than before. Now, any time I don't want to exercise, I remind myself that my numbers were consistently higher after exercise. Since I know that I am almost guaranteed to feel better, I am less likely to skip my workout.

Now, you might be thinking, "Making exercise a habit and eating well is easier said than done. How do I actually do that? The tips are all great, but how do I initially motivate myself to train enough times that working out becomes a habit? How do I motivate myself to make enough healthy nutritional choices that eating well becomes a habit?"

I get it. Knowing and doing are two very different things. I've found the following five motivational exercises very useful. I think number two is my personal favourite, but they're all great. Experiment and pick what works best for you.

### ⇒ Motivational trick 1

For the next two weeks, journal and rate your mood on a scale of one to ten before and after exercising. A rating of one means that you have intense negative feelings toward exercise and feel generally grumpy. A rating of ten means that you have intense positive feelings toward exercise and couldn't be happier. I've found that when people rate their mood between a one and

a five before exercise, it is normally six or above after exercise.

Another way of framing this same idea is the "law of initial value." That phrase has been etched into my brain ever since I took a psychology of exercise class during my undergrad studies. When applied to exercise, the law of initial value dictates that the worse you feel prior to exercise, the more opportunity there is for your mood to improve. Under this logic, the more unmotivated, cranky, or tired you feel before a workout, the more important the workout is.

Every time you want to skip your workout, remind yourself that your rating always improves after exercise.

### ⇒ Motivational trick 2

Use the "ten-minute rule." I love this rule. Basically, the rule means that even if you really don't want to work out, you have to make yourself do something, even just for ten minutes. Tell yourself that you have to do a minimum of ten minutes, but that if you still want to stop after ten minutes, you can. The rationale is this: Ten minutes of exercise is better than nothing, so if you do stop, that's okay. Usually, once you've done ten minutes, you'll continue and finish the workout. The next time you don't want to exercise, try it.

I credit this rule for getting me through ten marathons, over twenty half-marathons, seven half–Ironman triathlons (two-kilometre swim, ninety-kilometre bike ride, and a half-marathon), and one full Ironman (four-kilometre swim, 180-kilometre bike ride, and a full marathon). Endurance events are so long that they're daunting. I remember standing in the cold water in Lake Placid before my Ironman thinking, "How can I possibly do this? I should just quit and go back to bed." Instead, I

told myself, "Just start. Do ten minutes and if you still want to stop, you can." I didn't stop. Once I start a race, the crowds and the environment help to get me in the mood. At my half-marathon in Barbados I didn't want to start. I had myself convinced that the heat would make me have my worst race time ever. What happened? I got a personal best. I've come to learn that my pre-exercise mood is not a good indication of how well my race or training will pan out. I just never know how I will feel mid-workout. So it's always worth trying. If after ten minutes I want to stop, I can. I've only ever pulled out of one race. I used my ten-minute rule to make myself start — and I'm glad I started — but I was ill, and after ten minutes I knew it was not smart to continue. Starting was the right move because it allowed me

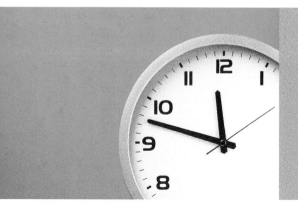

I even use this rule for writing. In fact, the ten-minute rule helped me write this book. Whenever I was unmotivated, I made myself write for a minimum of ten minutes. I told myself that after ten minutes I could stop if I wanted, but I never stopped. I usually ended up writing for at least two hours.

to make sure I was pulling out because of real illness, not just a bad mood. I have finished every other one of my races in large part because I used the ten-minute rule. It prevents me from feeling overwhelmed.

## ➡ Motivational trick 3

Make daily life your gym. This trick, like the ten-minute rule, is another way to make daily movement more palatable and less daunting. It concerns moving away from a conventional understanding of exercise. This is connected to my suggestion in chapter 1 of setting up a home gym and my suggestions in chapter 3 for how to weave movement into your daily life. Unless you are an athlete with very specific training goals, make your daily life your gym. When you frame your daily life as your gym, you will almost never have a legitimate excuse to skip a workout. Unless you have the flu, you literally can't escape the gym — it's all around you!

Gyms can be time-consuming to get to, and during the summer months it can be depressing to be indoors. Eliminating the act of having to get to a gym can make it much easier to make movement a non-negotiable.

Incorporate activity into your daily life: go for a walk with your partner at night instead of watching TV, use the stairs instead of the escalator, purposely take the long way to the bathroom, practise a sport with your kids, or even do some squats as the kettle boils or as you wait for the bus. Just move for thirty minutes a day. Don't feel like you have to go to the gym to get exercise. This way of thinking can be extremely useful on vacation. When you are away from home it is SO easy to simply say "Screw exercise; I am going to relax." Don't let yourself off the hook. Try a new sport like surfing, go sightseeing on a bike, or take a walking tour of the city.

## ➡ Motivational trick 4

Walk yourself through how you will feel depending on the choice you make.

When you want to skip your workout, first have a conversation with yourself. Talk yourself through how you will feel depending on the choice you make, and what type of person you want your future self to be. I love this. Other than the ten-minute rule, this is the motivational trick I use the most.

For example, let's say I want to watch TV instead of running. I first imagine how I will feel if I

When you have an urge to make a snap decision regarding your health, imagine how that decision will impact the rest of your day and your overall goal. Walk yourself through how you will feel three hours from now, and try to remind yourself of why you formed the goal in the first place.

accomplish my workout. I will feel great! My day will be better. The relaxation or social time I get to have after my workout (although possibly shorter) will be higher quality. I will be the version of Kathleen that I want to be.

I then imagine how I will feel if I skip the workout. I know I will feel crappy! I might get more time to relax, but the quality of the relaxation time will not be great. I will just sit there, metaphorically kicking myself, wishing I hadn't let myself off the hook. I will be annoyed at myself, because I will not be the version of Kathleen that I can be proud of.

On the flip side, if I am active, even if I just go for a twenty-minute walk, I will get less relaxation time, but I will enjoy that time more, and I will feel pride in my decision.

I am not arguing that you should never relax! Part of adopting a healthier lifestyle is building in time for yourself that includes adequate time to relax and sleep. I am not suggesting eliminating downtime. Instead,

schedule adequate sleep and relaxation time so that you can actually enjoy your downtime. Then move when you plan on moving. Get the best of both worlds — quality activity and quality downtime.

➡ Motivational trick 5

Last but not least, when all else fails, negotiate with yourself. Tell yourself you can have an extra-long bath if you lift weights or that you can listen to your favourite podcast only if you run. Or make a date with a friend and tell yourself that you can have coffee and a chat only if you have an exercise date first. When I am feeling unmotivated, I allow myself to buy a few passes for group-exercise classes at the new "It" studio. They are an added expense, but trying something new motivates me to train. Plus, I usually make a date with a friend to try the class since combining exercise and social time can be a great motivator. (I discuss the benefits of establishing what I call a health entourage in chapter 7.)

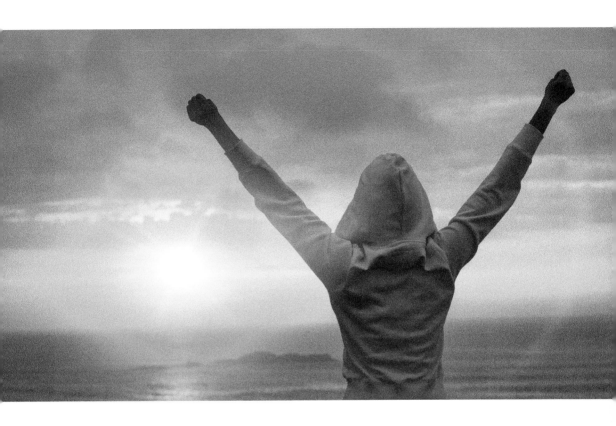

I am absolutely not above negotiating with myself. For example, I find bike intervals extremely difficult. (I do my intervals by placing my bike on a CompuTrainer — a stationary machine that measures watts, speed, and elevation). The intervals are hard. Sometimes when I don't want to do them, I make a deal with myself. I put my laptop on a bench beside my bike and watch TV during the recovery breaks between intervals.

# CHAPTER TAKE-AWAY

The next time you don't want to exercise, remember that everyone has moments of low motivation. Don't allow yourself to fall down the rabbit hole — the one where you convince yourself that you are the only person who struggles to exercise. That is not a helpful train of thought. We all have moments of low motivation; I know that I absolutely do. Remind yourself that you will feel better after the workout and that once you start exercising, it is easier to continue.

Get back on your fitness horse a more informed rider. Learn from your "down" moments. Maybe you don't want to exercise because your goals are unrealistic (see chapter 4), or maybe you are feeling discouraged because you are focusing only on the aesthetic benefits of exercise (see chapter 8). Whatever the reason, analyze the problem and persevere. Yes, the health journey is frustrating at times, but the struggle is worth it. The payoff is huge — it's your health!

Find activities that you enjoy or that inspire you. Sign up for a race. Train with a friend. Catch up on your guilty TV pleasures while on the treadmill. Or make your workout an adventure. Try a new running route or type of exercise class, or download new music. Reward yourself post-workout with a pedicure or a hot bath. Use whatever means necessary to make your workouts more fun, or at least more palatable. Tell yourself (sternly), "I am NOT the type of person who skips a workout." Working through these steps to set yourself up for success will mean that when you ask yourself, "When will I exercise?" the answer will be obvious.

# CHAPTER 3

# SOME MOVEMENT IS ALWAYS BETTER THAN NO MOVEMENT

Think of your daily health choices as drops in a bucket: small choices that seem meaningless, but which accumulate over time.

Some movement is always better than no movement may seem like a slightly obvious Kathleenism, and possibly even too basic to be useful, but don't dismiss the message as overly simplistic and, therefore, inconsequential. It is what I lovingly refer to as a "Captain Obvious" Kathleenism: well-known advice that still needs to be said since most people don't actually follow it. When it comes to health and wellness, the most obvious and boring solutions are usually the solutions people dismiss as irrelevant, but they are also usually the most helpful and economically accessible.

As I mentioned in chapter 1, we often set ourselves up for health failure by trying to find the perfect week to start training. Then when life takes over and we don't have time to complete the planned workouts, we allow ourselves to be inactive. When you live by the "some movement is always better than no movement" rule, regularly being active becomes more realistic.

Think about how many times in your life you have wasted opportunities to fit motion into your day or justified missing a workout because you didn't have time to get to the gym, do a full fitness class, or fit in a big run. The key word is

If you take away just one message from reading this book, make it "Stop aiming for health perfection. Just take every opportunity to move."

opportunity. You had time to be active, but you probably didn't think of the situation as a perfect opportunity for movement. Once you start looking for opportunities to move and reframing where movement happens, you will find that you DO have time to exercise.

Basically, don't use the fact that you can't get to the gym as a justification to be completely inactive. Find ways to weave motion into everything you do. Every bit of motion adds up and every situation can be reframed as an opportunity for movement. When you're feeling frustrated that the bus is late, smile and take it as an opportunity to walk. Forget something upstairs? No problem. Walking stairs is a great way to accumulate some steps. Had a bad day? No problem. Use it as incentive to go for a walk to clear your head.

Think some movement is always better than no movement.

Don't misunderstand me. I am not arguing that you shouldn't go the gym. If you can make it there, great. I love attending fun fitness classes and lifting weights. All I'm saying is, don't be a sloth when you can't get to the gym. If you have been wanting to adopt a healthier lifestyle for a while, don't use being in a "crazy-busy time at work" as an excuse to put it off. If you let it, life will always take over. So don't let it.

There is no perfect week to start training; just put on your running shoes and go out for a walk!

Part of my job is telling people things they don't want to hear — in this case, that you won't reach your health and wellness goals if you make healthy decisions only once every few weeks. Remember the two Cs of training: consistency and convenience. A workout can be touted as the most intense or "best" workout, but the best workout FOR YOU is the workout you will do on a regular basis. To achieve any health and fitness goal you need to be consistent, and the more convenient the workout, the more likely you will be to do it consistently.

Think of your health like a bucket. Every time you move, you accumulate water drops in your bucket. Small choices, like drops, accumulate over time. If you move regularly, your health bucket will eventually overflow, BUT (to paraphrase one of my idols, exercise and wellness guru Paul Chek) drops can just as easily evaporate. Basically, don't wait too long between bouts of activity. Your water droplets can evaporate. Accumulate drops regularly.

48    **FINDING YOUR FIT**

To accumulate your drops, think outside the "fitness box." Incorporate activity into your daily life. Bike or walk to and from work; learn to dance; go to your local park and train on the monkey bars; pace your office while on conference calls; explore the city with your family on foot; do some gardening. Or try working out at home (see chapter 11 for a detailed home program).

As I write this, I am envisioning receiving angry emails from readers telling me I am wrong to suggest they work out at home — that they love going to the gym and feel they couldn't possibly focus on working out at home. Many people feel they get a more focused workout outside their home. I get it. Fantastic. I am not arguing that you shouldn't go to the gym. If you can get to the gym, great. If you have found a method — any method — to stay active that works, then I say stick with it. Keep doing what works for you. As long as you are making DAILY (not weekly) movement a "non-negotiable," I am happy!

If you are thinking, "How exactly do I always do something? I am SO busy," don't worry. Use the following four strategies to fit movement into your busy life: "piggybacking," tracking steps, doing posture-friendly exercises throughout the day, and taking the colour challenge.

See chapter 11 for detailed exercise programs. There are five programs — each corresponds to a different exercise personality. If you identify with the information within this chapter (that is, if you are someone who knows they need to be active but currently has no time to get to the gym), look for an appropriate program under the heading "Time-Crunched Multi-Tasker Program."

# Four Simple Ways to Accumulate Your Drops

. . . . . . . . . . . . . . . . . . . . . . . . . . . . . . . . . . . . . . . . . . . . . .

1. Try the piggyback strategy. Instead of using "lack of time" or "I hate gyms" as an excuse to be inactive, pinpoint daily, non-negotiable habits that you already do and then turn them into a workout. I call this the piggyback strategy. Basically, the method just entails turning something you already do into a workout.

For example, turn your daily leisurely dog walk into a cardio workout by doing fartlek intervals. Fartlek intervals are challenging but unstructured, so you get a great interval workout without constantly looking at your watch. Warm up for five minutes, then pick a random landmark — such as a stop sign — and speed walk, run, or sprint toward it. Walk or jog to recover. Repeat until it is time to go home. Make sure to budget enough time for a five-minute cool-down.

If you usually take your dog to the dog park and throw him or her a ball, make your game of catch a strength workout. Do fartlek intervals until you get to the off-leash dog park. Once there, throw a ball for your dog. As he or she goes to fetch the ball, do body-weight exercises such as squats, lunges, burpees, or jumping jacks.

Try lunges as your dog races to get the ball.

## LUNGE

➡ Start standing. Step your right leg backward into a lunge. Keep both feet facing forward. Bend both knees so that your body moves toward the ground, then engage the bum muscle of your left leg to stand up. Make sure your front knee doesn't extend past your toe. Switch sides and repeat with the opposite leg. Aim for eight to twelve with each leg.

When you meet your goal, consider rewarding yourself with a predetermined non-food-related reward. Have a long bubble bath, take yourself to the movies, get a pedicure, buy a new workout outfit, or sign up for a new, fun "fitness adventure" like a dance class.

Other ways to use the piggyback strategy

- Instead of doing work or wasting time on your phone as you sit waiting for your child to complete her after-school activity, bring your exercise clothes and use that hour to go for a walk or run. If you want to watch your child's practice or game, do squats and lunges on the sidelines. Or bring a mat so you can do floor work. You could even bring a resistance band; wrap the band around a tree to do a set of rows. Or do bicep curls — hold one end of the band in each hand, let the middle of the band rest on the floor so you can step on it. While anchoring the band with your feet do a bicep curl by bending at your elbows to pull your hands toward your shoulders.
- Pace while on conference calls.
- Get up regularly and walk to your colleagues' desks instead of phoning them.
- Brainstorm for work while walking; dictate your thoughts into your phone.
- Instead of meeting with colleagues and eating or drinking, walk and talk.

2. Take the daily step challenge. An easy way to incorporate movement into your life is to record how many steps you take daily. I ask most of my clients to record their daily steps with a pedometer. Their initial recordings are typically around 2,000 or 3,000 steps per day. That is the equivalent of moving only one kilometre throughout your ENTIRE day. Unfortunately, that is fairly typical. Too many of us go from our home to the car, then to our desk, then back to our car, and drive home to sit in front of the TV.

Desk jobs may be a necessary evil, but complete inactivity throughout the day doesn't have to follow.

My clients are living proof. By simply changing small daily habits, most of them are now clocking 10,000-plus steps per day and are feeling way more energetic and fit.

The trick is to make sure you progressively increase your steps. On day one, wear the pedometer or use the tracker on your phone, but don't actively try to take more steps than usual. Record how many steps you take. Use that number as your baseline. SLOWLY increase your steps — your tissues need time to adapt. It is not uncommon to develop negative pain in your joints, feet, or back when you increase your steps too quickly. Increase your daily step count by 1,000 steps per week until you are at 10,000.

My clients rose to the occasion, and so can you. You just have to take the time to plan HOW you will fit your steps in. You can't just

## Simple ways to get your steps

- Go for a walk at lunch with a colleague.
- Get off public transit a stop early and walk to your destination.
- Park a couple of blocks away from your destination.
- Walk with your partner after dinner.
- On the weekends, walk while doing your errands.
- Constantly "forget" something in another part of your home — preferably on another floor.
- Set an alarm to go off once an hour to remind you to get up and walk around. Get water or go for a stroll around the office.
- Turn on some music and dance around your living room or do some jumping jacks.
- Run or walk the stairs in your home or apartment building.
- Practise a sport with your kids; throw the softball or football around.
- Play an active game like hide-and-seek with your kids.
- Get your partner or neighbour committed to getting 10,000 steps per day. Use that other person as motivation. Call each other or email every night to check in and make sure you both have gotten your steps.

Try challenging yourself to make 10,000 steps per day a non-negotiable. By that I mean that if you get to the end of your day and are only at 9,000 steps, find a way to fit in another 1,000 steps. Don't go to bed or relax on the sofa until you have fit in those steps.

wish them into reality. You need a plan of action.

Now for the fine print. Don't let yourself off the hook if you walk or run daily in a structured way for exercise. Aim for 10,000 steps in addition to your structured workouts. The idea is to build movement into your daily life. Don't get me wrong — going to the gym is GREAT. If you can get there, go for it, but in addition to going to the gym, try to subtly change your lifestyle so that you sit less and move more.

**3.** Do posture-friendly exercises throughout your day. Another way to accumulate your health drops is to pepper simple posture, strength, core, and balance exercises into your day. Even doing just a couple of exercises at your desk every day will make a difference. I suggest prioritizing what I call "posture-friendly" exercises because most of us sit too much, which results in poor circulation, headaches, bad posture, and often stiffness and pain. Posture-friendly exercises are any exercises that stretch

out the chest and improve upper back, neck, and core strength. Just because you have a desk job doesn't mean you are destined to slouch and have upper-back discomfort. You don't have to live with discomfort! You just have to become more aware of your posture, and strengthen and stretch your neck, upper body, and core.

Now, I know, the head and neck are not the most glamorous body parts to train. Getting nice legs or a toned tummy is often what motivates people to work out, but being aware of posture is important. A forward head (when the head migrates forward) can cause a cascade of negative effects — the most tangible being pain and discomfort. Possibly more important, it leads to poor posture.

The human head is typically between thirteen and twenty pounds. When twenty pounds consistently pulls your body forward, the upper back and neck have to work to compensate for the extra weight. (Imagine if you had to hold twenty pounds straight out in front of you for a prolonged period. Think how

# POSTURE-FRIENDLY EXERCISES

I had originally branded these as "posture-perfect" exercises until a very wise friend said that using perfect didn't mesh with my philosophy. She was right. So don't aim for posture perfection. Instead, conceptualize these exercises as movements that will help you trend positive in the posture department. Here are a few of my favourite posture-friendly exercises. More examples can be found in the program section of chapter II.

**Wall push:** Stand with your back against the wall, knees slightly bent, arms straight, and palms facing the wall. Your palms should be gently touching the wall, but don't get distracted by your hand placement. The motion is about moving your shoulder blades. Yes, your hands will push slightly into the wall, but only because your shoulder blades and your upper back are initiating the motion. Pull your shoulder blades back, tuck your chin like you are trying to give yourself a double chin, and simultaneously push into the wall with your hands. Don't let your lower back arch as you pull your shoulders back into the wall. Hold for five seconds. Release and repeat ten times.

**Door-frame chest stretch:** Place the forearm of one arm against the edge of a door frame at roughly chest height. Your arm should be bent at a ninety-degree angle. Turn your body gently away from the arm so that you feel a slight stretch in your chest and shoulders. Hold for thirty seconds. Switch and repeat with the opposite arm.

**Seated twist:** It is almost impossible to have good posture if you can't rotate properly. Extension of the spine (the ability to sit up straight) and rotation work together. Sit tall in your chair. Reach your left hand across your body so that it sits on the outside of your right knee. Use your left hand to pull GENTLY on your right knee so that you rotate to the right. Hold for fifteen seconds and then switch sides.

**Seated core work:** A strong core will help you maintain proper posture. Start by bringing your bum close to the edge of your chair. Keep your back straight and lean backward roughly ten degrees. Hold for ten seconds to a minute.

## Upper-back massage with a tennis ball: All you need is a tennis ball and wall space. Stand with your upper back against the wall, with the ball between your back and the wall. Press your body into the ball so that you feel a gentle massage. Move your body up and down so that the ball massages your entire back. When you feel a tender spot, hold and breathe into it for ten seconds. Enjoy!

## Wall Ys to Ws: Stand with your bum and back against a wall, core engaged, legs shoulder-width apart, knees slightly bent, and feet roughly half a foot in front of the wall. Your lower back should be neutral, which means you should be able to fit your fingers, but not your entire hand, between your lower spine and the wall. Form a W with your arms against the wall. Keep your arms as close to the wall as you can while you straighten them until they form a Y with your body. Make sure that your spine stays neutral. It shouldn't arch as you move your arms, even if that means the back of your hands move away from the wall. Return your arms to the W position and repeat five to ten times.

## Shoulder, elbow, arm rotations: This exercise has three parts. Start with your arms straight and by your sides. For part one simply roll your shoulders backward. For part two lift your elbows up as you roll your shoulders back. Meaning, lead with your elbows. Your elbows should move backward behind you as you roll your shoulders. For part three, keep your arms straight as you make a big circle backward. In this move your hands will reach backward. Try to feel your shoulder blades move as you do all three actions. Repeat the cycle five times.

## Figure-four stretch: Sit tall with your shoulders back. Look straight ahead as you cross your right ankle over your left knee. Push gently on your right thigh. Feel the stretch in the outside of the right hip. Hold for ten to thirty seconds and repeat on the opposite side. Don't allow your body to rotate toward the leg that is being stretched. Keep your shoulders stacked over your hips and your hips and shoulders level side to side. Meaning, your right shoulder and your right hip should not be higher than your left shoulder and left hip, and vice versa. If you are wearing a pair of exercise pants with the coloured stripe around the waist, the strap would be parallel to the floor, making a horizontal line. It would not be tipped in one direction.

Has your head been "sucked forward" by various screens? Test yourself. Have someone look at you from the side. Stand naturally. Don't cheat by moving your head back. Get them to drop an imaginary line from your ear downward. The line should fall roughly in line with your shoulder.

exhausted your arms would be. When your head sits forward, your upper back and neck are under a similar type of strain.)

If your head sits forward, please DON'T try to jam it backward. That can cause different but equally problematic postural imbalances. Postural habits take years to develop; they can't be reversed in a day. The first step in reversing forward head syndrome is to be aware of the problem. The next step is to carefully do something about it.

Regularly get up from your desk. (Bonus: this will help you accumulate your steps.) Try to move around at least once an hour. Get water, walk around, and do a few posture-friendly exercises.

Also, get an ergonomic assessment of your workspace. Make sure your computer, chair, and desk are at an appropriate level and that your computer is straight in front of you, not off to the side. See if your boss would consider investing in a standing desk for you. If not, no problem; try using a filing cabinet to set up a makeshift standing desk for yourself. A few times per day, stand up to do work at your desk. Whether you are sitting or standing, think of orienting yourself backward. This will help you gently bring your head back without

## FOUR-WEEK POSTURE-FRIENDLY PROGRAM

WEEK I: Challenge yourself to do one posture-friendly exercise between breakfast and lunch, and one between lunch and the end of your workday.

No excuses! Two exercises per day is nothing. Set an alarm if you need to!

WEEK 2: Challenge yourself to do one posture-friendly exercise between breakfast and lunch, one at lunch, and one between lunch and the end of your workday.

Make these exercises non-negotiable. Tell yourself that you can't have your mid-morning and afternoon coffee or tea break, or your lunch, before your exercise is done. Posture-friendly exercises take about a minute. No matter how busy you are, you always have a minute.

forcing the movement and causing other problems.

If you are confused about how to start introducing posture-friendly exercises, don't stress. Try my four-week program.

4. Take the colour challenge. Use a mindfulness trigger (a colour) to cue yourself to be aware of your posture and do some movement.

Let me explain. First, pick a colour to use as your mindfulness trigger. Next, pick what the trigger will remind you to do — tailor the trigger to fit your day.

If it is a weekday, and your job is fairly formal, use the colour as a reminder to assess your posture. When you notice your colour, check if your ears, shoulders, and hips are stacked over top of one another. If your body is not aligned properly — which is the case for most of us — sit or stand up straight to gently draw your shoulders and head back.

On the weekends, take it up a notch. Decide that when you see "red" you will assess your posture, but when you see "blue" you will do a few jumping jacks or one of the posture-friendly exercises.

If you work from home, decide that every time you see the colour you will walk up the stairs once.

You can even use the colour as a reminder to drink water.

Once you have picked your colour and what activity you will do when you see it, watch for your chosen colour throughout your day. When you see it, do your chosen activity.

You can be as creative as you want with this challenge. The world is your fitness oyster!

WEEK 3: This week, I want you to start taking these posture-friendly exercises more seriously. Try to average one every hour and a half. Again, set an alarm if you need to. Ideally, piggyback one positive health choice onto another. When you stop to do a posture exercise, also drink some water.

WEEK 4: By now, doing posture-friendly exercises throughout the day should feel fairly natural. So let's up the ante. Your final challenge is to do one posture-friendly exercise per hour. Here's the kicker: Don't just do one exercise an hour this week. Aim to do one exercise an hour every workday from now on.

# CHAPTER TAKE-AWAY

Always remember that your health quest is something you are doing for YOU! Adopting a healthier lifestyle is about self-care. Care enough about yourself to make daily movement a non-negotiable.

You don't need to spend money and energy investing in every new miracle workout program. Captain Obvious health solutions — like walking more, doing fartlek intervals, and building a home gym — may not seem flashy or innovative, but they are the inexpensive cornerstones of long-term health and an easy way to live by the rule that some movement is always better than no movement.

# CHAPTER 4

# MAKE FITNESS GOALS, NOT FITNESS WISHES

If you don't plan exercise in advance, it usually doesn't happen.
Book exercise into your schedule like any other appointment.

"I am going to start working out next week."

"Come Monday, the gym will be my new best friend."

"After tonight, no more junk food."

"This year is going to be different. I am going to work out and lose weight."

These types of unrealistic declarations are examples of what I call fitness wishes. Wishes are like hoping someone will wave a magic wand and make you healthier.

Now, I am guilty of having expressed many fitness wishes in my life. Who hasn't? I am not saying, "Don't wish." Wishes have their place; they can be a great first step, but actually adopting new, healthier habits or losing a significant amount of weight, and then keeping it off, requires a long-term approach.

Without a concrete implementation plan, these wishes will most likely be forgotten as soon as you get busy. Grand health statements are too easy to dismiss. Whatever my ambitions, I achieve them only when I take the time to establish realistic fitness goals and a corresponding plan of attack.

The trick to making your fitness wishes come true is to establish realistic, safe, and sustainable long- and short-term goals. Basically, you need to learn how to make goals, not wishes.

# Six Steps to Making Goals, Not Wishes
## (abbreviated version)

**STEP 1** Stop using the "I am too busy" excuse; you may be too busy to get to the gym, but you can always find ways to be active.

**STEP 2** Don't aim to change all your health habits at once. Prioritize your goals! You can't overhaul your entire lifestyle overnight. Decide which lifestyle changes are realistic and will have the most impact on your health. Then make these changes your key goals.

**STEP 3** Establish both long-term and short-term goals. Breaking goals down into smaller, more manageable pieces can help you avoid feeling overwhelmed.

**STEP 4** Respect your genetics. Don't waste your life wanting to look like a celebrity or be a waif if you don't have those genetics; tailor your goals to fit your genetics, your age, the current realities of your life, and your current fitness level. Aim to be the best and healthiest version of yourself that you can be.

**STEP 5** Form goals that are relevant and important to YOU. Don't exercise just because your doctor or spouse tells you it is healthy.

**STEP 6** Learn from yourself and others. Learn from your successes, as well as your less-than-ideal choices. Learn from others, then implement any strategies that speak to you and your lifestyle.

# Six Steps to Making Goals, Not Wishes (detailed version)

· · · · · · · · · · · · · · · · · · · · · · · · · · · · · · · · · · · · · · · · · · · · · · · · ·

## Step 1 Stop using the "I am too busy" excuse

"I don't have time" is the grown-up equivalent of "the dog ate my homework."

Okay, I know that if you are not a fitness professional, whose job it is to be fit, training can't (and shouldn't) always take first priority. Other aspects of life, such as work and family, often need to be prioritized, but the quote highlights that too often people use lack of time as an excuse for abandoning their health goals — a way to downplay the need for self-reflection, mindfulness, and realistic, structured goal setting.

Being "too busy" is a "no-analysis-needed, get-out-of-exercise-jail-free card." It is used to — either consciously or unconsciously — disregard real logistical or emotional impediments standing in the way of adopting a healthier lifestyle.

So, if you justify being inactive because you are "too busy," take a moment to ask yourself, "What is really going on?" You may be busy, but are you really too busy?

**Have you unconsciously or consciously structured your life so that your needs always come second?**

If you are actually that busy, why? I doubt that you can't find even ten minutes to go for a walk, but if you really can't, maybe that tells you something about your priorities. How, and possibly why, have you consciously or unconsciously structured your life so that you have no personal time? Are you too busy because you put the rest of your world's needs ahead of yours? I work with many parents who are willing to give up everything for their kids. I respect that they are such great parents, but I always tell them, "Adopting a healthier lifestyle is about self-care as well as about being a positive role model. You have to care enough about yourself to put healthy food into your body and carve out time to be active. Being healthy will ultimately make you a more vibrant and present parent or partner. Actively caring about your health is also a way for you to model healthy behaviour for your family. I am not suggesting you neglect your kids; I just know that there are ways to be a fantastic parent and be good to yourself at the same time." Think of it like the oxygen mask on an airplane. Parents are instructed to put their masks on first; they will be of no help to their kids if they are unconscious on the floor.

If you are too busy to get to the gym, incorporate movement into your daily life. Consider the piggybacking strategy I mentioned in chapter 3; piggyback activity onto things you already do. Do squats and lunges as you watch your children practise their sport, walk your kids to school then jog or run home, or pace as you take conference calls. See chapter 3 for more ideas or read chapter 11 for a detailed program.

### Do you use the "I am too busy" excuse because you are trying to commit to a plan you hate?

At least at the beginning, don't say you will run five days per week if you hate running. If you hate something, you will always find other, more "important" ways to use your time. Instead, make exercise palatable. Make a date with a friend — I love trying different fitness classes with my friends and then going for tea after. Or sign up for adult dance classes. My friends and I have taken several dance classes together, including salsa lessons and a two-hour "learn to dance like Britney" workshop.

### Do you lean on the "lack of time" excuse because you have a strict, uni-dimensional definition of exercise?

Redefine how you understand "exercise." As I discussed in chapters 1 through 3, understanding exercise as only going to the gym or going for a run is not always helpful. When life gets in the way, it is easier to abandon health goals altogether and say something like, "Since I can't do my full workout, I don't have time to work out at all." Can't get to the gym? No problem. Do some weights in front of the TV (for a detailed program you can do in the comfort of your living room, see chapter 11), go for a walk at lunchtime, or climb the stairs in your office building. Make movement, not exercise, a non-negotiable. Sure, a full gym workout may be the ideal, but the benefits are moot if you can never achieve the ideal.

### Are you "too busy" because you are afraid of failure and don't want to try?

"I don't have time" is so easy to say, and since there is often a kernel of truth to it, being "busy" allows us to disengage with our real emotional relationship with our bodies and exercise.

Be honest with yourself about WHY you didn't exercise. Own your choice.

For example, sometimes people say they are too busy when really they are — consciously or unconsciously — afraid that failure is inevitable, so why even try. I have witnessed others who use the "too busy" excuse because their current internal self-image doesn't quite mesh with the image of the healthy person they want to be. Yes, part of them wants to be healthier, but a larger part of them can't actually imagine themselves as a different person. So it is easier to be busy then admit the truth and work through those feelings.

Don't sabotage your health efforts. Take the time to reflect and be mindful about your health choices.

### Are you "too busy" because you haven't taken the time to rearrange your schedule?

Preparation, preparation, preparation. Of course you are too busy to work out if you haven't carved out the time. Schedule in your workouts and analyze your upcoming week so you can troubleshoot possible problems and come up with solutions. For example, if you schedule a weekly Tuesday run with a friend, look at your work schedule in advance and see if you have possible conflicts. Either fix your work schedule or, if that is not possible, email your friend and reschedule the workout. Don't wait until Tuesday morning to realize you are going to have to skip the run.

The main take-away is this: Stop letting yourself off the hook by using the "I am too busy" excuse. Be honest with yourself. If you hear yourself using time as a justification to abandon a health goal, take a moment to reflect on what is really going on. Work through any emotional barriers that might be keeping you from following through on your health and fitness goals. Set a realistic goal, take the time to analyze how you can schedule training into your life, and troubleshoot possible setbacks in advance. It will probably take you a while to work regular training into your life — that's okay. Just get the process started. If you decide that you legitimately don't have time to do a structured workout like a fitness class, instead of abandoning your goals altogether, simply work more movement into your daily life.

**Step 2** Don't aim to change all your health habits at once. Make realistic, specific goals and establish a detailed plan of action

Establish two or three realistic goals; they should reflect the time and energy you actually have (not how much you want to have), your finances, and your equipment. Figure out in advance the WWWH of your workout plan.

**W:** WHERE and WHEN will you work out? Will you join a gym and go before work, join a running group, set up a home gym, or play a sport? Take into consideration what you like to do, how much time you can dedicate to your training, what you can afford, and what is convenient.

**W:** WHAT exercise will you do? Plan to do something you actually enjoy, or at least something you don't hate. If you love being outside, research the local ravine system or find a nature walking group. If you love group sports, find a convenient team to join. If you know you need help being accountable, get a fitness buddy (see chapter 7 for details).

**W:** WHEN do you want to accomplish your goal by? Be specific. If you want to lose weight, how much and by when? Break the goal down — how much per week? If you want to get stronger, what exactly does that mean? Do you want to be able to do more push-ups? If so, how many and by when? Make sure your time frame is realistic.

**H:** HOW will you fit in your training? What accommodations do you need to make? Do you need to rearrange who will drive the kids to school? Do you need to block off time during your workday? Do you need to download fitness podcasts or buy DVDs so you can train in your living room? Do you need to arrange child care so you can train after work?

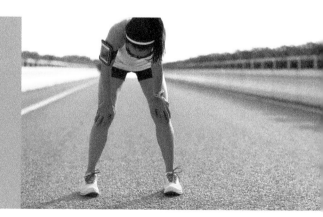

Don't set yourself up for failure by aiming to change all of your health habits at once.

Your WWWH plan should be specific. For example, instead of saying, "I am going to work out," say something like, "I am going to meet my friend at the gym three times a week after work. When I have evening work events, I will take a walk at lunch."

Instead of saying, "I am going to lose twenty pounds," say, "My goal is to lose one to two pounds per week for ten to twenty weeks. I am going to do this by walking to and from work, bringing my lunch daily, and refraining from eating sweets."

After you have established your goals and specific plan, ask yourself, "How will I stay on track?"

Regardless of how amazing the plan is, know that there are going to be moments when it is hard to stay committed; situations — like parties — where you don't have complete control can be challenging. It is unrealistic (and frankly unhealthy) to say that you are never going to go to parties or end up in other such tempting situations. Go, but acknowledge in advance that the situation will be tricky and figure out a plan of attack. Offer to bring a salad so that you have something healthy to eat, or copy me by never hanging out near food. That way I can't mindlessly nibble. I will discuss various "health danger zone" management tricks in chapter 6,

but the main take-away is to identify potential danger zones in advance and make a plan.

Last, make yourself accountable; write down your goals and share them with your friends and family. Note why the goals are important. Whenever you want to abandon them, read over the reasons and remind yourself of why you initially formed the goals.

## Step 3  Establish both long- and short-term goals

Breaking goals down into smaller, more manageable pieces can help you avoid feeling overwhelmed. For example, if your long-term goal is to lose twenty pounds, a possible short-term goal would be to lose one pound per week for a total of twenty weeks.

I establish both yearly goals and monthly goals. For example, my 2013 goal was to improve my cycling so I could achieve a personal-best racing time. To accomplish my long-term racing goal, I committed to doing bike intervals eight times per month. The intervals helped me strengthen my legs, which in turn allowed me to achieve my long-term racing goal.

For the longest time, I could not make myself floss daily. Every time I went to the dentist, I felt frustrated and guilty because I knew flossing was not that hard or time-consuming, but I still couldn't make myself do it.

I decided to apply the techniques I teach my clients to my oral health: I gave myself the strict (but caring) talking-to that I would have given one of my clients. I told myself to stop feeling guilty because guilt would just make me want to pout, or worse, continue to be a negligent flosser, just to show my dentist who was boss. I told myself to ditch the guilt and self-pity and instead to implement a plan of action.

So, game on! I established my long- and short-term flossing goals.

My long-term goal: Improve the health of my gums by making flossing a regular part of my daily routine.

My short-term goal: Floss every day for one month.

Brainstorming past and future roadblocks is something I encourage my clients to do, so I decided to brainstorm why my past attempts at flossing had failed. I decided I had failed at flossing in large part because I always planned to floss when I brushed my teeth, but that was unrealistic because I am too rushed in the morning and too tired at night.

I decided I would incorporate flossing into an already established midday routine. (I call this piggybacking — see chapter 3.) Since I exercise and shower daily, I decided that I would floss after exercising and before showering. I left floss at work and in my backpack so that it was always available.

I now floss regularly (mostly). Go me! When I fall off the flossing wagon, which I do once in a while, I assess why and then get right back on track. The same goes for exercise. If you make a goal that you don't stick to, don't worry. Assess why you did not succeed and then create new goals based on your new-found knowledge.

## Step 4 — Respect your genetics, the realities of your life, your current fitness level, and your age

"Respect your genetics" may sound obvious, but in my experience, most of us don't. Our goals are often grand, unrealistic, and non-specific. Our desires have been clouded by exposure to both mainstream media and information within the fitness field.

Let's use fitness magazines as an example. Grand weight-loss promises — like "Lose twelve pounds this month!" — are ubiquitous in health and fitness magazines.

Statements like this imply that everyone can, and should, lose twelve pounds this month. News flash — it is not a safe or realistic goal for everyone to lose twelve pounds of weight in one month. That is three pounds per week. The closer you are to your ideal weight, the harder it will be for you to lose three pounds per week. A heavier man may easily lose three pounds per week, but a smaller woman will have a hard time losing that much. This is especially true if she has already lost a considerable amount of weight or has always been at a healthy weight.

The amount of weight you need to lose depends on how much weight you have already lost and how close you are to a healthy norm. Popular fitness discourse often makes it seem like we all need to lose ten pounds, but not everyone has ten pounds to lose. Factors that will influence how much weight you can and should lose are your age, your gender, your metabolism, and your past weight-loss history. You might not even need to lose weight. Maybe you need to gain muscle. Or maybe you have already lost weight and to lose another twelve pounds would be unhealthy.

All weight loss is not created equal. The faster the number on the scale decreases, the more likely the weight you are losing is muscle or water, not fat. It is challenging and time-consuming to lose fat. Muscle and water are easier to lose, but their loss will not change your body shape as drastically. In addition, when you lose muscle your metabolism decreases, which makes it more likely that if you put the weight back on you will replace the lost muscle with fat, which simply makes it harder to lose weight in the future. Plus, rapid weight loss can cause health complications including weakening of the heart muscle, irregular heartbeat, and dangerous reductions in potassium and electrolytes. For long-term, sustainable weight loss, I usually recommend that my clients aim to lose between half a pound and two pounds per week. Care about fat loss, not just the number on the scale!

Plus, if you initiate your health quest with unrealistic expectations, these unachievable goals will make it impossible for you to succeed. When you don't reach your goals, a negative domino effect can occur. You may just revert to the unhealthy habits you were trying to move away from.

Embrace who you are! Don't waste your life wanting to look like someone else or have somebody else's arms. Stay in your own health lane; aim to be the best and healthiest version of you that you can be. Don't expect that exercise will give you Serena Williams's body if you are five feet tall and one hundred pounds soaking wet. I will never be a world-class marathon runner. I don't have the genetics or the time to dedicate to the sport. If winning a marathon were my goal, I would constantly feel like a failure. I should, and do, have athletic goals, but I set my goals within realistic parameters. Training for a sub–four-hour marathon is realistic for me. Aiming for a sub–three-hour race, or to win an Olympic weightlifting competition, is not.

Take it from me. I hated being tall as a teenager. I spent years wanting to look like anybody but me. Those negative thoughts were such a waste. I should have been enjoying those years, not judging myself. I will never get my teenage years back.

Basically, set yourself up for success by setting realistic goals that are based on your own body. Don't compare yourself to your friend, a celebrity, or even your mother.

Don't get caught up in fitness challenges — like the "squat challenge" — that promise generic results. Sure, do some squats — squats are a fantastic functional exercise — but squatting does not produce the same results on every body. An individual's age, gender, activity level, genetics, nutritional habits, and fitness and health history affect how they will respond to any exercise program. Unless you are monitoring your food, doing additional forms of exercise, and/or have excellent genetics, simply doing squats will not aggressively change your body or make you look like the model in the ad. Plus, you don't become fit by doing any one single exercise. Sure, squats are great, but only when done in conjunction with other exercises.

*For years I set unambitious racing goals because I was afraid to fail. This meant I never reached my racing potential. Now I try to set realistic yet challenging goals so that I have something to work toward. If I don't succeed, I try to learn from my mistakes and train smarter for my next race.*

## Step 5 — Form goals that are important and relevant to YOU

We all know that exercise is good for us. The doctor might be able to scare us into exercising for a week or two, but knowing the scientific benefits is often not enough to make working out a priority over the long term.

Part of successfully adopting a healthier lifestyle long term is finding reasons to exercise that are relevant to YOU.

Let me give you an example: It is scientifically true that a twenty-year-old female swimmer should lift weights to ward off future risk of osteoporosis, but osteoporosis is probably not relevant to a twenty-year-old. She might acknowledge the scientific truth that swimming is a non-weight-bearing activity and thus doesn't help to dramatically improve her bone density, but it probably won't motivate her to actually lift weights if she would rather just be in the pool. For her, she might need to be told that strength training will improve her racing times.

I know that when I was fifteen, if someone had told me I had to do exercises

to improve my posture I would have just rolled my eyes. Now, at thirty, I am more motivated to strengthen my posture. I can see that biking has caused my shoulders to round forward, and I don't like it.

Yes, make realistic and specific long- and short-term goals, but the more you can connect your goals to something you care about — or as I said in chapter 2, your WHY — the more likely you are to follow through on them.

Aim to stretch so you can hang out with your grandkids on the floor, or strength train to prevent injuries. Just establish goals that mean something to you and make sure that you have the ability to follow through on them.

## Step 6 — Learn from yourself and others

Learn from yourself. Each week take the time to reflect on what you did well and areas that need improvement. Use journaling as a way to form a positive internal dialogue; be proud of your accomplishments. Figure out how you can reproduce positive

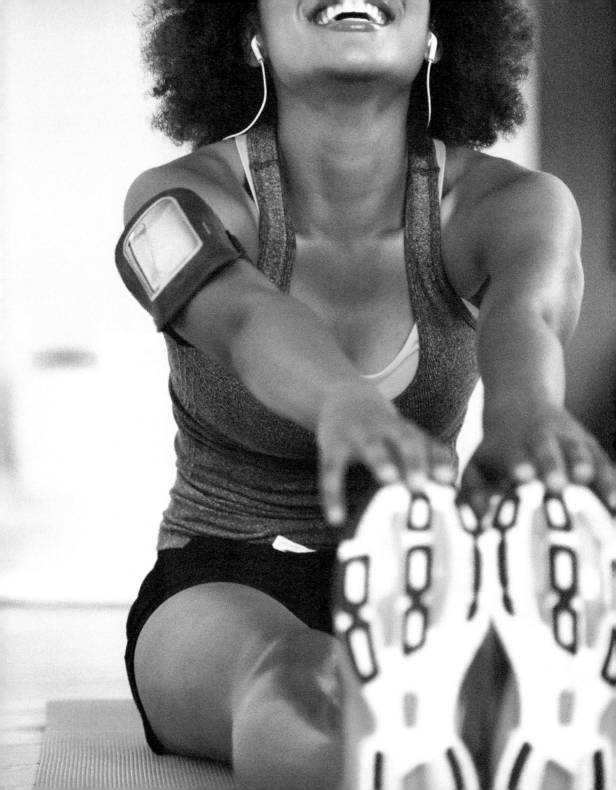

health choices, and learn from choices that you are not proud of.

Learn from others. Talk with your friends and read the relevant literature. Check out credible websites such as PubMed (www.ncbi.nlm.nih.gov/pubmed), the Healthy Living Zone from Bandolier, Oxford (www.medicine.ox.ac.uk/bandolier/booth/booths/hliving.html), Bandolier's Knowledge Library (www.medicine.ox.ac.uk/bandolier/knowledge.html), the Mayo Clinic's healthy lifestyle section (www.mayoclinic.org/healthy-lifestyle), MedlinePlus from the U.S. National Library of Medicine (www.nlm.nih.gov/medlineplus), and Health Canada's food and nutrition and healthy living resources (www.hc-sc.gc.ca/fn-an/index-eng.php and www.hc-sc.gc.ca/hl-vs/index-eng.php). I am also a huge fan of anything published by health expert Paul Chek (chekinstitute.com). For full workouts and exercise descriptions, check out my Pinterest page (www.pinterest.com/KTrotterFitness). Basically, research what has worked for others, then implement any strategies that speak to you and your lifestyle.

For example, a 2005 article in the *American Journal of Clinical Nutrition* states that there are four characteristics shared by people who successfully lose ten percent or more of their body weight and maintain that loss for at least one year:

➡ They exercise daily (that obviously makes me, an exercise enthusiast, very happy).
➡ They are diligent about monitoring their diet, calorie intake, and weight.
➡ They eat breakfast.
➡ They don't cheat on weekends or holidays.

Through research and trial and error, figure out what works for you. Find YOUR own recipe for success. Play around. You can't implement everything you read or every strategy that worked for your friends and family; advice is not useful if it isn't relevant to your life. Acknowledge what others are doing, but don't get caught up in their health journey. Be picky and strategic — decide to implement only strategies that speak to you and your lifestyle. Stay in your own health lane!

# CHAPTER TAKE-AWAY

Set attainable goals that are based on accepting yourself for who you are. How your body responds to exercise will be influenced by your age, gender, genetics, fitness history, nutritional habits, and current activity level.

Don't keep your goals a secret. Tell your friends and family what you want to accomplish. Stating the goal out loud, so that other people know about your plans, can help keep you on track. Write your goals down. Writing your goals down will help you be more accountable to yourself.

Remember, health is a lifelong process. I tell myself that my "end goal" is simply to always be consciously moving toward a healthier version of myself. The key words being *lifelong* and *moving*; health is not a linear process. It takes daily dedication. You won't wake up tomorrow and miraculously be "healthy"; think big picture. Adopting a healthier lifestyle is not just about making one change, such as not eating bread. Gradually, you want to work toward a time when you sit less, move more, and are more mindful of your daily nutritional choices. Learn from any missteps and persevere.

# CHAPTER 5

# ADOPTING A HEALTHIER LIFESTYLE IS A MARATHON, NOT A SPRINT

Keep this well-used Kathleenism in mind: When you fall off the "health horse," don't give up. Use it as a learning experience and get back on a more informed rider.

When I was growing up, my mom always stressed the importance of managing expectations. She taught me that managing my expectations — of other people, myself, and situations — is paramount to my own happiness. I try to apply this life lesson to everything, including my understanding of health and wellness.

Applied to health and wellness, "managing expectations" is shorthand for "embrace the fact that adopting a healthier lifestyle is a marathon, not a sprint, and to survive the marathon, you need to change your attitude."

If you expect your health journey to be a marathon that includes periods of higher and lower motivation, you are less likely to throw in the towel when you make a misstep.

Too many of us buy into the myth that you can lose weight quickly, and then keep it off easily.

Stop thinking that you should be able to change your lifestyle and body overnight. Unhealthy habits take time to form. Healthy habits are no different. Recalibrate your expectations and understand that making healthier choices is something you are actively choosing to do, not something that is being forced upon you. Appreciate that you have the ability to participate in the journey. Always learn from your mistakes and persevere.

Take a moment and contemplate how often you set yourself up for weight-loss and health failure by expecting results that are simply not possible to achieve, let alone maintain.

Basically, "buy in" for the long haul.

To do this you need to learn how to change your attitude toward exercise. Notice that I used the word learn. As I stated in chapter 1, adopting an active lifestyle is a conscious and active process. Embrace the marathon and recognize that to survive it you have to change your attitude toward health. Adopting a healthier lifestyle is all about having the right attitude.

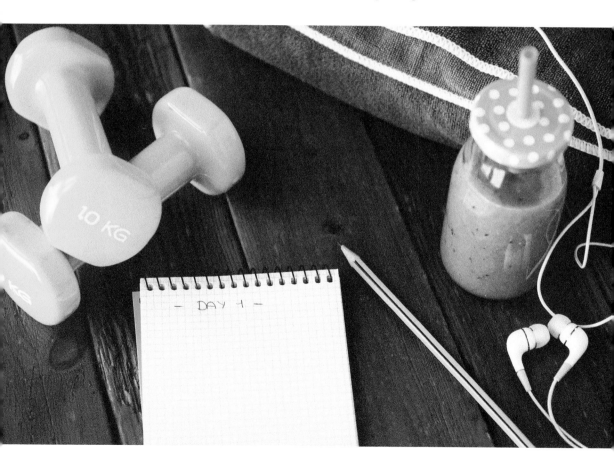

## How to Change Your Mindset Toward Health and Wellness (abbreviated version)

**STEP 1** Understand that you have the power to modify your response.

**STEP 2** Find opportunities to be positive; concentrate on what you CAN do and CAN eat instead of what you CAN'T do or CAN'T eat.

**STEP 3** Stop seeing exercise as something that you are being forced to do. When you frame health as something being imposed on you by others, the have-to-ness of exercise and eating well often makes them feel suffocating and stressful. Instead, understand exercising and eating well as choices.

**STEP 4** Make your positive health choices create a domino effect; consciously make them bleed into and affect the rest of your life.

**STEP 5** Reframe setbacks; use mental and physical hurdles as opportunities for growth and learning so that you can make better choices in the future.

**STEP 6** Aim to trend positive. We all have days that are healthier than others. What changes is what we consider a healthy day to be. Have more healthy habits this month than you had last month so that you slowly find a new, healthier normal.

**STEP 7** Stay in your own lane. Your health process is exactly that — your health process. Don't get caught up in what your friends and family are doing. Don't let anyone else's choices dictate your choices. Be your own health boss.

**STEP 8** Stop judging yourself and others. It is counterproductive. The fear of being judged can be debilitating and often becomes yet another barrier to being active.

**STEP 9** Have a personal mantra prepared (your SIU — "suck it up" lecture); when needed, use it to give yourself a stern talking-to.

# How to Change Your Mindset Toward Health and Wellness (the detailed version)

. . . . . . . . . . . . . . . . . . . . . . . . . . . . . . . . . . . . . . . . . . . . . . . . . . . . . .

## Step 1 Understand that you have power

Realize and embrace that you are not destined to always feel oppressed by exercise, or to always feel unhappy that you have to move.

You have the power to modify your response to exercise and healthy eating. Renowned psychologist Viktor E. Frankl said, "Between stimulus and response there is a space. In that space is our power to choose our response. In our response lies our growth and our freedom." Now, I am sure he wasn't referring to exercise, but I find the application extremely useful.

Think of the stimuli Frankl refers to as all of the food and exercise options available to you. Learn how to modify your response to these stimuli. Instead of understanding eating well and exercising as something that is constraining you, understand being able to move as something that is enjoyable, something you get to do. Embrace the joy of exercise.

## Step 2 Find opportunities to be positive

Concentrate on what you CAN do and CAN have instead of what you CAN'T do or CAN'T have! Embrace the privilege of moving and eating well.

I tried modifying my response while racing the 70.3 Ironman in Mont-Tremblant. (A 70.3 consists of a two-kilometre swim, a ninety-kilometre bike ride, and a half-marathon.) Every time a negative thought came into my head — such as, "I am not fast enough" or "My feet hurt" — I tried to flip the thought. I replaced the negative thought with a positive one such as, "The scenery is so beautiful," "I am so thankful to be injury-free," and "I did all the training I could possibly do, so now all I can do is give it my best." I ended up getting a personal-best time and, more important, I had one of the most enjoyable racing experiences of my life!

I started thinking about the importance of finding the positive after a client injured her foot and couldn't run for roughly six months. Now she can run again and she is SO grateful; she always glows when she talks about her runs. One of the reasons she enjoys running is that she frames it as a thing she "gets" to do. Our conversation solidified my belief that to successfully become healthier in the long term, we all need to focus on what we can do and what we can have instead of focusing on what our body can't do or what we can't have.

Replace "I have to exercise" with "I get to move."

In my experience, most of us frame health and wellness around deprivation — becoming healthier ends up being about the cake you can't eat and the social activity (like drinking) you have to cut out. No wonder so many people don't stick with their exercise and healthy-eating plan. Who wants to feel constrained as well as deprived of what they love?

The thing is, if you have ever been injured, you know just how much of a privilege moving can be. The few times I have been injured were such wake-up calls. I missed running. Now, whenever I don't want to run I remind myself of when I couldn't run and I really wanted to. Instead of feeling constrained by having to run, I have learned to embrace the fact that I can run.

The key word is learned. I wasn't born knowing how to embrace movement. I taught myself how to see the positive. As I said in chapter 1, adopting a healthier lifestyle is an active process. Part of the process is actively relearning how to frame movement — finding ways to flip your feelings. Focus on what you can do and what you can eat, not what your body can't do or what you can't eat. Turn negative thoughts into positives.

Basically, you have to find the positive.

Instead of "I can't eat cake," think, "How great is it that I can eat these delicious berries?"

Instead of "I don't want to go for a run," think, "How lucky am I that I can run?"

Instead of "I can't have seventeen beers," think, "I am going to have one glass of wine and enjoy it and then be able to feel great tomorrow and be productive when I wake up."

Instead of "I don't want to stop sleeping," think, "How great is it that I will get to run on the sidewalks before the rest of the city wakes up?"

Learning to embrace the positive is not easy. Believe me, it is a lesson that I have had to learn over and over again, but it is a lesson that is worth at least trying to embody.

# Step 3 Stop seeing exercise as an imposition

Move away from adolescent resistance toward health and wellness. Part of finding the positive is moving away from understanding exercise as something that you are being forced to do, and instead understanding it as a choice. When you frame healthy choices as something imposed on you by others, they become just more things on the to-do list. This have-to-ness of exercise often makes it feel like something that is imposed, suffocating, and stressful, which for many of us, makes us revert back (often unconsciously) to a childhood feeling of someone telling us how we "should" behave. We all sometimes metaphorically stomp our feet at authority, say, "Screw it," and choose to eat ice cream. Asserting control becomes connected to having that extra glass of wine or sleeping in.

Move away from this adolescent resistance to adopting a healthy lifestyle. If you have some ice cream, don't feel guilty. Enjoy the ice cream. If you decide that you weren't happy about the choice, learn from the mistake and make a better choice next time. Own the choice. You are an adult. Appreciate that you have the power to decide to eat ice cream, and you also have the power to make a different choice next time.

# Step 4 Make your positive choices create a domino effect

Focus on the positive choices you make. Let your positive choices bleed into the rest of your life.

Let's say you want to skip your entire workout but instead you convince yourself to do half. Actively concentrate on the fact that you did something, not on the fact

When I started running, all I wanted was to be able to run a sub-2:15 half-marathon. I thought that would make me a "real" runner. When I reached that goal, I decided I wanted to run a sub-two-hour half-marathon. I repeatedly changed my goal — I would accomplish the goal and then I would simply change the criteria in my head. That meant I was never fully happy with my accomplishments. I never let myself think of myself as a real runner. Don't get me wrong: establishing new goals is an important aspect of fitness. I am proud of myself for making and accomplishing my athletic goals. But I am not proud that I let forming new goals detract from the initial pride I felt in my achievements. We all (myself included) have to learn to value the process of working toward goals, not just of achieving them. I will not stop setting athletic goals, but I will try to live in the present and enjoy being a runner as opposed to thinking of what I will feel like when I accomplish my next goal.

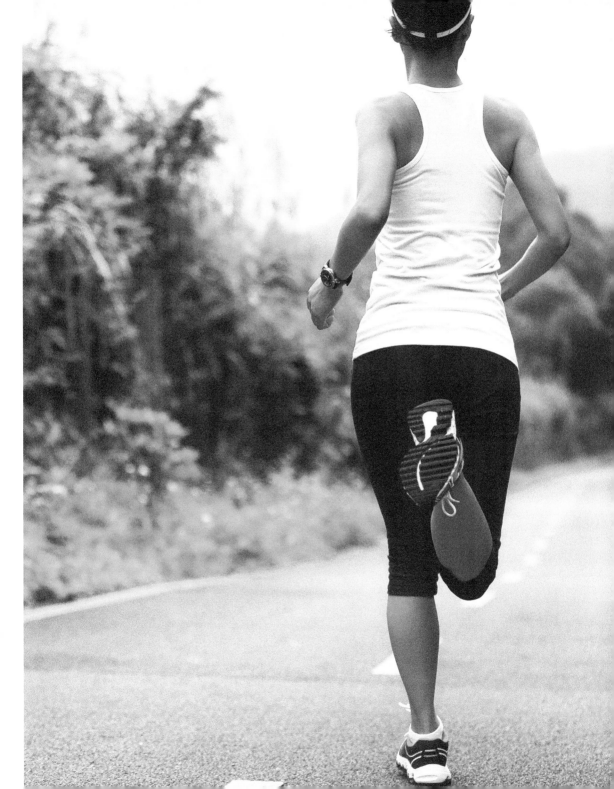

that you didn't do the entire thing. Create a positive domino effect so that you continue to make positive health choices.

If you make positive choices bleed into the rest of your day, your inner dialogue will hopefully sound something like, "I wish I had done my entire session, but I am proud of myself for doing something. If a partial workout made me feel good, my entire workout tomorrow will make me feel great."

If you let a negative dialogue bleed into the rest of your life, you risk an inner dialogue that sounds something like, "I am such a failure. I am never going to be fit. I might as well eat that bag of Doritos."

To be clear, I am not arguing that you should pretend you made ideal health choices if you didn't, or take an "Oh well, who cares" approach. Instead, I am suggesting you become mindful and respectful of yourself. Find the positive in what you did do. This will allow you to replicate positive choices, and will hopefully propel you to have a generally more positive day. Plus, this approach allows you to learn from your choices instead of being dragged down by them.

# Step 5 Reframe setbacks

Setbacks are inevitable, so learn from them.

As I said at the beginning of this chapter, adopting a healthier lifestyle is in large part about recalibrating your expectations. If you expect your health journey to be a marathon that includes periods of higher and lower motivation, you are less likely to throw in the towel when you make a less-than-ideal health choice.

Setbacks, like those that might occur at a party, at a wedding, or after a break-up WILL happen.

Instead of using setbacks as an excuse to abandon your goals altogether, reframe the experiences; expect and embrace them. Mental and physical hurdles are an opportunity for growth — an opportunity to learn how to make a better choice next time. As I said in chapter 1, learn to flip your thoughts. When you make a choice you are not proud of, own that choice and then figure out why you made it (were you tired or depressed?) as well as how you can make a better choice next time.

Each week, reflect on what you did well and areas that need improvement. Figure out how you can reproduce your positive health choices. Make a list of less-than-ideal choices you made and figure out how you can avoid them. Anticipate future roadblocks, and find solutions in advance.

When you find yourself struggling to follow through on your goals, instead of being discouraged, remind yourself that you are not alone. The further you get

For a few months in 2014 I seriously debated breaking up with running, which was a big deal. Running is my happy place. Whether I am single or committed, lighter or heavier, moody or tired, running puts a smile on my face. When clients or friends told me that running made them feel awkward or tired, I listened, but I didn't really get it. Since I didn't remember the frustrations associated with starting to run, I didn't truly understand how running could be anything other than wonderful. Then in February and March of 2014, I didn't run. The weather was terrible and running is hard on the body, so a break seemed like a good idea. Taking a running hiatus is — in theory — healthy, but my mood suffered. I was noticeably crabbier without running — especially at first. So I figured that my first run back would feel amazing. It didn't. On April 1, I laced up my shoes with excitement. Instead of feeling awesome, I just felt awkward. Running was hard in a way I didn't remember. I actually started to think that maybe instead of pushing through the terrible initial phase of running, I should just take up another sport. Thankfully, I did push through. I gradually got back into the swing of running. My love returned. So, if you are having trouble learning to enjoy exercise, know that you are not alone. Finding the motivation to exercise, to push past any initial awkwardness, to find your exercise bliss, is a challenge. Health is a process. Getting into a routine takes time and patience — even for a trainer! Recalibrate your expectations. Expect that adopting a healthier lifestyle will take long-term dedication. That way, you can embrace health hurdles instead of letting them defeat you.

from the start of any goal, the harder it can become for most of us (including myself) to stay on track. Instead of spiralling into a negative domino effect of unhealthy choices, start by reminding yourself of why you initially established the goal, and that every day, not just New Year's Day or your birthday or September first, is a good time to adopt healthier habits. If you have fallen off your "health train," don't wait until the next milestone to get back on. Start again NOW. Resolve to keep on trying (and trying and trying). Adopting a healthier lifestyle is a long, time-consuming, and often frustrating, but ultimately highly rewarding, process.

## Step 6 Aim to trend positive

Try to abandon the "good" versus "bad" binary classification that often accompanies the quest for weight loss and improved health. As I suggested in chapter 2, aim to trend positive; aspire to have more healthy habits this month than you did last month. We all have some days that are healthier than others. What changes is what we consider a "healthy" day to be. A healthy day is relative to your normal. Have more healthy habits this month then you had last month so that you slowly find a new, healthier normal. I still have chocolate once in a while, but it is no longer an everyday occurrence like it was when I was fifteen. My normal has changed and now consists of tons of vegetables, lean protein, and healthy fats.

You didn't establish your current health habits overnight, so give yourself time to learn to enjoy exercise and develop a taste for healthier foods. Aim to gradually create healthier preferences — gradually being the key word. Health is a long-term process. Think of your health like the stock market. Expect ebbs and flows — just ensure that the general trend is upward.

## Step 7 Stay in your own lane

As I mentioned in chapter 2, your health process is exactly that — your health process. Don't get caught up in the trendy diets your friends are trying. When you go out to eat with friends or family, don't let their choices dictate your choices. Be your own health boss, stay in your own

Find opportunities to be active instead of excuses to be sedentary.

lane, and, whenever possible, surround yourself with people who will support the new and healthier you.

# Step 8 Stop judging yourself

Judgment becomes yet another barrier to being active!

Being watched when working out might be exactly what some people desire, but for many the fear of going to the gym and being looked at with a critical gaze can sap any will to exercise. What is worse is that often individuals internalize this critical gaze: we all become our own worst critic. The fear of being judged can be debilitating. I work at a private studio so people don't have to be looked at by other members when they are working out. Many of my clients tell me that although they will train with me, they don't want to go to their local gym on their own until they start to look fit. Many clients have even told me that they put off hiring a trainer because they did not feel fit enough. They were worried about being judged by the trainer — this is a great example of how judging oneself and others is counterproductive. As I mentioned in chapter 1, judgment too often keeps people from actually starting or maintaining a workout

program. Anxiety over achieving a certain "look" (versus just becoming fit) and self-criticism usually become yet more barriers to becoming active.

I want people to stop being so worried about looking fit. It is not useful. Our fitness goals should be about becoming fit and energized. This is especially true for me. It is easy for me to get caught up comparing myself to other trainers and feeling like I have to model perfect, healthy habits for my clients. The reality is that we are all human, and fitness and health involve a lifelong learning process, not an end result.

Basically, open the door, step outside, and just move!

# Step 9 Have a personal mantra prepared

When needed, use your SIU — "suck it up" lecture — to give yourself a stern talking-to.

Setbacks may be inevitable, but that doesn't mean I think you should constantly let yourself off the hook when you make an unhealthy choice. Just because it is possible to learn from unhealthy choices doesn't mean you have a built-in excuse to make them.

"Adopting a healthier lifestyle is a lifelong process" is not code for "put off, till

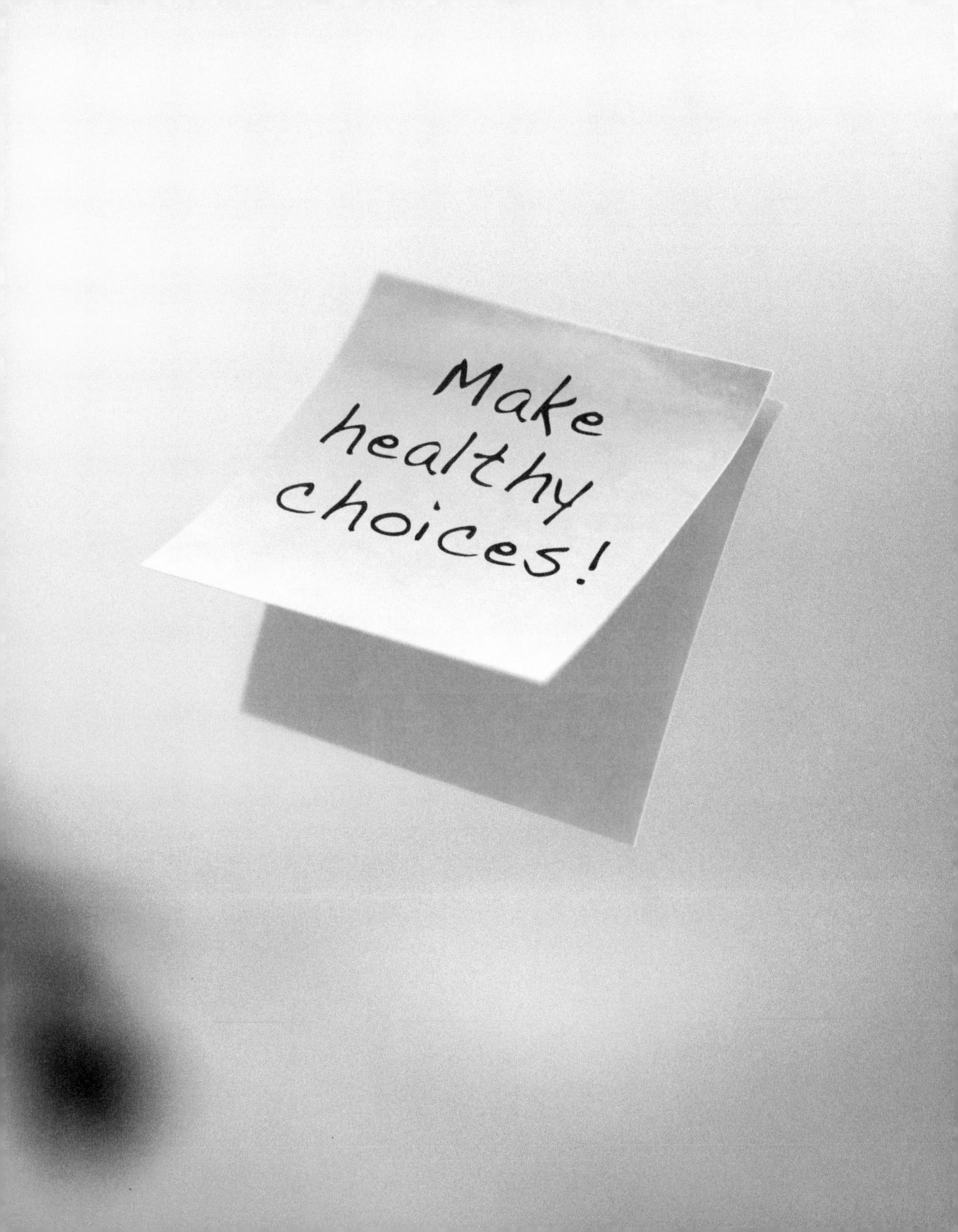
Make healthy choices!

tomorrow the healthy choices you can make today."

When I don't want to train, my SIU lecture sounds something like, "Kathleen, you ARE the type of person who works out. You always feel better after a workout. Movement is a non-negotiable. Just do something, even for just ten minutes."

Prepare yourself. You are not a robot, so adopting a healthier lifestyle will be hard work — you will have to give yourself a few SIU lectures. That is to be expected. Until you change your health habits, norms, taste buds, and internal health dialogue, making healthier choices will take mindfulness and dedication. Prepare yourself to do a few things you don't absolutely love.

I am not talking about making yourself eat something you hate or you are allergic to, or doing a workout that will injure you, but if there are healthy foods you are ambivalent about, like broccoli or kale, sometimes you should just choose to eat them over the unhealthy option you love. Or at least eat more of the healthy option.

Part of adopting a healthier lifestyle is finding the balance between short- and long-term satisfaction. Make yourself eat the healthy foods you don't love (short-term pain) so that your taste buds evolve and you learn to appreciate your greens (long-term satisfaction and health). This is especially true at the beginning. You need to change your taste buds and health habits so that you create a new health normal.

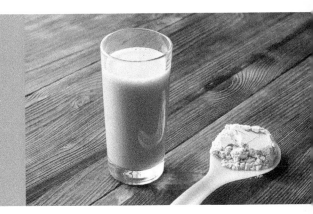

I often have clients tell me things like, "I don't like protein at breakfast." My answer? "So? Protein is important. Find a form you can tolerate." The point is that as long as you are not allergic to a particular food, sometimes you just have to learn to tolerate healthy options.

# CHAPTER TAKE-AWAY

Have realistic expectations. Setbacks will happen; be prepared and don't let them derail your progress. Learn from the experience. Aim to trend positive, and persevere. Expect your health journey to be a marathon that includes periods of higher and lower motivation — embrace the marathon!

At the beginning, it is hard to make yourself be active or eat your greens, but once you are used to it, it feels weird to not move and eat your vegetables. Health is a process. Part of that process is finding the balance between instant satisfaction and long-term success. Putting up with a short-term annoyance is a small price to pay for health, happiness, and satisfaction in the long term. Obviously, everyone's goals and daily realities are different, thus this balance will differ from person to person. Find the balance that works for you. If you don't succeed initially, keep trying.

Health is not a linear process — aim to have more healthy habits next month than you did this month.

Remember that your health quest is something you are doing for YOU. You are a grown-up deciding to be good to yourself. Try to revel in how wonderful it is that you can eat healthy foods and exercise. Eating fresh berries is a present to yourself, not a punishment. Deciding to eat processed crap full of preservatives is not a reward.

Adopting a healthier lifestyle is about self-care. Care enough about yourself to put healthy food into your body.

# CHAPTER 6

# FIND THE WWHH OF YOUR EATING HABITS AND ADOPT THE CAPTAIN OBVIOUS APPROACH TO HEALTH

To successfully change your eating long term, you need to figure out not just WHAT and HOW MUCH you eat, but HOW and WHY you eat.

Stop trying to find the "perfect" diet to follow. When you follow a predetermined diet or exercise plan — one that is not individualized, reflective, or intuitive — it is too easy to fall off the program and revert completely back to old, unhealthy habits.

More important, since the causes of weight gain are multifaceted and vary from person to person, what causes weight loss will also vary person to person. Our eating habits are tied to our emotions, our established habits, our lifestyle, and our childhood eating habits.

Work toward finding the WWHH of your eating habits: WHAT you eat, WHY you eat, HOW you eat, and HOW MUCH you eat.

The operative word here is YOU — ditch the cookie-cutter approaches to weight loss. Explore your unique relationship with food; pinpoint your trigger foods and situations, and the nutrition and exercise habits you most need to improve on.

Do you eat when you are tired? Sad? Angry?

Once you have analyzed your health habits, you won't need the dogmatic rules of any diet or to rely on an expert's knowledge to make healthy choices. You will have the tools to follow your own

If modifying your exercise and nutritional habits at the same time is too overwhelming, start by changing only one. Remember the Kathleenism from chapter 3: Some movement is always better than no movement. Don't let the goal of "health perfection" paralyze you and stop you from moving forward. Try walking more. Then gradually modify additional habits. Simply aim to have more healthy habits this month than you did last month.

personalized plan, grounded in what I call the Captain Obvious principles of healthy eating — universal nutritional habits that transcend the boundaries of any one diet. These include stopping eating when you are full, drinking water, and eating more vegetables.

If you are currently following a program, and it is working for you, great. Keep at it. Adopting a healthier lifestyle can be overwhelming — having a program to follow, especially at first, can be helpful. Health is a process. I ask only that you make sure the program is based on healthy principles (so, no extreme diets), and that as you follow the program, you also work on becoming mindful of not just WHAT and HOW MUCH you eat, but of HOW you eat your food and WHY you eat.

You can overeat out of boredom or sadness on any diet — SkinnyPop Popcorn, mangos, and low-fat pudding might be "allowed" on Weight Watchers, but nothing is "skinny" if you eat multiple portions. Don't fall into the trap of believing that finding the "perfect" diet will ensure that you will reach your health and fitness goals. You need to change your mindset. Sure, an intelligent plan can be a helpful jumping off point, but if you don't become aware of your personal WWHH patterns, you will simply continue to fall off your health horse or find the loopholes in every plan you follow. Ultimately, being successful is not about the plan you chose to follow, but your mindset. The plan will only work if you have a healthy and productive mindset. Don't transfer responsibility on to any one plan — your "health buck" stops with you.

# WWHH —WHAT, WHY, HOW, and HOW MUCH You Eat

Most traditional diets and nutrition regimens primarily focus on WHAT you should eat and/or HOW MUCH you should eat. Both elements are obviously invaluable — no one is going to adopt a healthier lifestyle or lose weight if they are eating large portions of fast food daily. But you should also start being mindful of HOW and WHY you eat.

Really, the key word is not what, why, or how, but you. Identify your personal danger zones, habits, and triggers. Whether it is late-night eating, social nibbling, fast food, or alcohol, the key is becoming mindful of your habits. Once you pinpoint your habits and trends, you can find appropriate solutions.

Trying to change too many things at once can be overwhelming, so figure out the nutritional habit that is having the biggest negative impact on your health. Fix that first. Choose the habit that will give you the most bang for your habit-changing buck.

Once you see the difference created by one positive change, it will be easier for you to make other positive changes. I call this the "positive domino effect."

Main take-away: If you need structure, follow a set program (for now), but also become mindful of not just WHAT and HOW MUCH you eat, but more important, of HOW and WHY you eat. If you don't address the WWHH of your eating habits, your personal food habits will follow you from nutrition program to nutrition program.

Ask yourself the following four questions:

What do I eat?

■ Do I eat fast food? Prepared foods? Foods high in sugar or saturated fats?

Why do I eat?

■ Because I am tired? Sad? Angry? Am I a social eater? Do I eat when nervous or when I am trying to please someone? Or do I eat more when I am alone?

How do I eat?

■ In front of the TV? Too quickly? Standing up? Do I pick off my partner's or kids' plates? Do I nibble off my co-worker's desk?

How much do I eat?

■ Do I eat adequate portions? Always go back for seconds? Am I always stuffed after a meal? Do I snack even when I am not hungry?

# How to Become Aware of the WWHH of Your Eating Habits

## Strategy | Keep a food journal for two weeks

Use it to pinpoint the WWHH of your eating habits.

The basic concept: Record food choices and portions as well as alcohol and water consumption for a set period. Then analyze your nutritional choices and patterns.

Before my clients start to journal, I ask them what percentage of their diet they think is made up of healthful choices. For weight maintenance, I suggest that 80 percent of the diet be healthy choices. For weight loss, roughly 90 percent should be healthy.

Clients generally tell me they follow the 80/20 or 90/10 rule, but usually after we analyze their journal we find that they have been underestimating the unhealthy choices they make and overestimating the number of healthy choices they make.

There is often a disconnect between the choices people think they are making and the choices they are actually making. Keeping a journal can help highlight the disconnects.

There are two variations that I like even more than the traditional journal.

The "X versus O" journal offers a bird's-eye view of your nutritional habits, not simply of your particular food choices. Draw five big circles on each page of a journal (these circles are the Os referred to in the title). Each page represents one day of eating. The five circles represent three meals and two snacks. After every meal, ask yourself, "Did I stop eating when

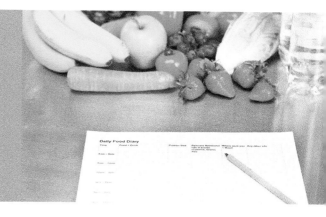

Keeping a journal can often work as a slight self-correcting mechanism — people tend to dislike having to write down what they consider less-than-ideal choices. So, consciously stick to your usual diet for a week. That way, you will be able to analyze your usual patterns and work to find appropriate solutions.

I was full, and did I generally make healthy choices?" If the answer is yes, simply put an X through the appropriate circle.

If you made food choices that you were not happy with, write in the circle WHAT you ate, as well as HOW much you ate, HOW you ate the food, and WHY you ate the food. Were you tired or depressed? Did you grab food mindlessly off your co-worker's desk or eat in front of the TV?

At the end of a week, look over your food journal. Hopefully, your week will be full of Xs. If the Os have been filled in, figure out when and why you made your unhealthy choices. Learn from your choices. Figure out how can make better choices next time.

In the "hunger versus want" journal, instead of writing down what you ate, simply note the level of your hunger and degree of fullness before and after each meal. Before each meal, write down if you ate when you were ravenous, hungry, full, or stuffed. After each meal, write down if you stopped eating when you were pleasantly satisfied, full, or stuffed. Use this data to learn in which situations you overeat.

You may be inadvertently sabotaging your efforts by making what I call "unhealthy healthy choices" (hence why journaling is key — it can highlight counterproductive choices).

Clients usually don't need me to suggest they cut out sweets and fried foods. The fact that foods like chocolate bars and french fries are unhealthy is fairly common knowledge. Obviously, actually cutting out sweets and fried food is hard work, but knowing they need to be eliminated (or at least reduced) is usually a no-brainer.

When a client journals that they ate something like ice cream, they are aware that they made the choice to have a treat. I obviously suggest portion control or alternative options, but in general, they don't need me to point out the potential health problems of that choice.

It is the less obvious culprits — the unhealthy healthy foods — that tend to slide under the radar and inadvertently sabotage progress. There are two categories of unhealthy healthy food.

The first category consists of foods that are high in sugar and/or salt that masquerade as health foods. Basically, these are wolves dressed in sheep's clothing. Think store-bought muffins (just cake in the shape of a muffin), juice (liquid sugar), most store-bought granola (sugar and fat), frozen "healthy" dinners (preservatives and salt), most gluten-free desserts (just because they don't have gluten doesn't mean they are healthy), many restaurant-style salads (dressing, cheese, bacon bits), and fat-free snacks (usually devoid of nutrients and full of artificial crap).

The second category consists of foods that are very healthy in moderation (as in, if you eat one or two portions), but that are not healthy when consumed willy-nilly. Think almonds, peanut butter, crackers, and high–glycemic index fruits (mangos and pineapple). This second category is especially significant for people who want to lose weight. The key to weight loss is not only food selection but also portion control. Too often, when you know that something is healthy, you might be less mindful and not worry about portion control.

Side Note: the glycemic index is a ranking of foods from 0 to 100 based on their immediate effect on the body's blood sugar levels. Basically, the number is a measure of the speed at which your body digests the food and converts it to glucose. The faster the rise in blood glucose, the higher it will rate on the index. In general, one wants to aim to have the majority of their diet from foods with a lower glycemic index. Foods with a lower glycemic index include most vegetables, berries such as raspberries and blueberries, nuts and seeds, beans and lentils, and low glycemic index grains such as bulgar, oats, and basmati (not ordinary white or brown) rice. Lean meats and poultry contain no carbohydrates so they have no GI value.

Copious amounts of almonds (which, yes, are more nutrient-dense than copious amounts of potato chips) are not part of a nutritionally balanced day. Handful after handful of nuts is not helpful to your health quest, especially if one of your main goals is to lose weight.

Again, yes — an apple with almond butter is a great snack, but not if you are consuming over 500 calories of almond butter a day during your afternoon snack. For an average size woman, 500 calories is not a snack.

Don't misinterpret my words — I am not suggesting that you might as well eat seven pieces of chocolate cake. Obviously, blatantly unhealthy foods like doughnuts are still unhealthy. What I am saying is, be mindful of what, how, and why you eat. A gluten-free cookie can be made of as much crap as a regular cookie. No matter what you are eating, portion control is key. Don't stand at a party or at your kitchen counter and snack mindlessly. Sit down and enjoy what you are eating. If you decide to have an amazing piece of cake, great. Enjoy your treat. Just have one small slice, not seven.

Do you mostly eat because you are hungry (a biological need)? Or do you eat when you are still full because you "want" food? Wanting food is more of an emotional than a biological response to food.

Too many people stop once they have collected their data. The point of keeping a journal is not simply to get the data, but to analyze the journal and learn from it. For example, I have learned that I make bad food choices when I get too hungry or too thirsty. Armed with this knowledge, I always ensure that I have a water bottle and a healthy snack with me so I don't stop and impulsively buy chocolate or arrive home starving and gorge on everything in sight. If I want chocolate I have chocolate, but I do it mindfully, in a way that I know my "future" Kathleen will be proud of.

## Strategy 2 Reframe the WHY

Instead of thinking of food as the enemy or as a reward, or of eating as something to do when you are tired, happy, sad, or angry, think of food as fuel and of eating well as self-care. Choose to eat well because you love yourself and to fuel your brain and body.

Fill up on foods that pack a nutritional punch. Aim to eat the foods that have the highest nutritional density possible — vitamins and minerals help your body to produce vital hormones and neurotransmitters, stabilize blood sugar, provide energy, increase your body's ability to repair itself, and help you sleep. Don't starve yourself or try to exist on low-calorie, nutritionally empty low-fat foods like rice cakes or zero-fat yogurt.

As an athlete, I am motivated to eat well because a well-balanced diet drastically improves my mood, performance, alertness, and energy level. A healthy diet can be the difference between a personal best and a personal worst.

When you want to grab something like a muffin out of convenience, remind yourself that juggling work, family, and social obligations is your athletic feat of the day. Life is hard on the body; everyone should fuel like an athlete because everyone needs to perform at their best. A healthy meal can be the difference between a productive, energy-filled day, and a midday sugar breakdown.

## Strategy 3 Use my "thirty-minute rule" and my "party five" trick

Teach yourself to take a beat between the moment you want a sugary, salty, unhealthy treat and the moment you eat it.

At home: wait thirty minutes. Don't tell yourself you can't have the treat you're craving; that will make you feel deprived and will possibly make you binge. Instead, tell yourself (preferably out loud) that you can have it later, if you still want it. Do something — wash the dishes, play a board game — anything that will keep you busy. Usually after thirty minutes, you will no longer want the treat. If after thirty minutes you decide you are legitimately hungry — versus tired, bored, or sad — have a healthy snack like some vegetables and a tablespoon of hummus. If you feel like you absolutely need the actual treat, have a very small portion.

At parties: use my "party five" trick. Have some water, get involved in an interesting conversation with someone far away from the food table, and consider how you will feel if you consume the treat. If after five minutes you decide you have to have it, go for it; just enjoy a moderate portion. Life is worth living; eat a moderate portion and make sure you choose a treat you really love. Don't eat things you don't truly love.

Move away from needing a prescriptive diet. Learn to listen to your body, and adopt the Captain Obvious principles of healthy living — principles that transcend "diets."

You don't have to spend tons of money on cleansing programs, protein powders, or the latest miracle food to achieve your health and wellness goals. I am not saying don't eat goji berries (or this month's equivalent miracle food), I am just saying that adopting a healthier lifestyle shouldn't be about eating (or not eating) one particular food. Instead, learn to listen to your own body and become mindful of your unique habits and triggers.

You don't need to spend oodles of money or follow a restrictive diet, you just need to get back to basics.

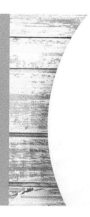
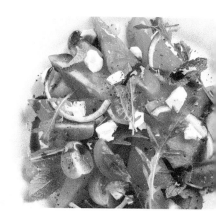

A simple, yet effective goal is just to move more this week than you did last week. The more you move around, the less time you spend sitting.

I was a vegetarian for roughly eighteen years, until about 2013. In 2013 I asked myself why I had become a vegetarian. The answer? Becoming a vegetarian allowed me to assert my independence, feel in control, and separate myself from my parents. At age twenty-nine, I realized that I didn't want my health decisions to be reactive. I decided to start eating meat so that I could assess if the older, grown-up version of Kathleen wanted to become a vegetarian again. It was time to re-evaluate the decision of the eleven-year-old version of me. After all, if I still lived by all of my eleven-year-old choices, I would only watch movies with actors like Fred Astaire and Gene Kelly, and only wear clothing that reminded me of Judy Garland.

I am not saying that everyone should eat meat. I am also not making a moral or ethical argument regarding being a vegetarian. I am still in the process of figuring out what the adult, health-conscious Kathleen should eat. What I do know is that whenever possible, I am now aware of why I am choosing a particular food, and of how much I am consuming. This awareness is what I hope to instill in my clients and anyone who reads this book. There is no magic diet or magic food. Lifelong healthy eating requires awareness and an understanding of your own emotional relationship with food.

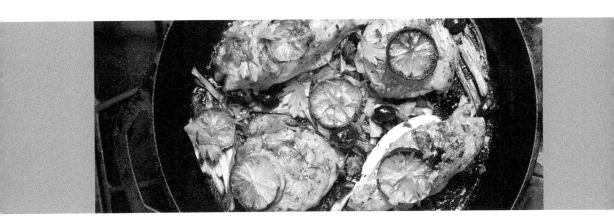

# The Captain Obvious Principles

· · · · · · · · · · · · · · · · · · · · · · · · · · · · · · · · · · · · · · · · · · · · · ·

## Principle 1 — No matter what you are eating, stop when you are full

Don't eat just for the sake of eating. You don't have to finish everything on your plate. Stop eating when you are satisfied. Don't wait until you are stuffed to push away your plate.

Don't use the rules of your nutritional regimen as a way to justify eating foods in a way you know is not healthy or helpful. For example, just because you are "gluten-free" doesn't mean you should eat ten gluten-free cookies. Or if you are on Weight Watchers, don't scam the system by eating seven pieces of fruit just because they are "free." In Weight Watchers, every food has a point value, and you get to eat a certain number of points daily. Most fruits and vegetables are considered zero points, or "free," to encourage users to choose fruits and vegetables over foods like french fries. I think this is great, but if you have eaten all of your points and you are full, listen to your body and stop eating.

Portions count. If you have had enough, stop. Period. No exceptions.

## Principle 2 — Don't eat mindlessly

Before you put anything in your mouth, take what I refer to as a "mindfulness moment"; ask yourself if you are actually hungry and if your future self will be happy with your choice. If your future self won't be happy, or if you are actually bored or sad, step away from the food.

- Don't eat while standing — for example, while socializing at a party or cooking.
- Don't eat in front of the TV or computer.
- Don't eat while you are working or while walking.
- Put your fork down in between bites. Don't hoover down your food. Slow down and savour the flavours. Enjoy your meal and the company you are with.

Don't assume that just because you have heard this Captain Obvious advice a million times you are actually following it. When it comes to health and wellness, the most obvious and boring solutions are usually the ones people dismiss as irrelevant, but they are also often the most helpful and economically accessible.

## Principle 3 Chew your food

Paul Chek taught me the phrase, "You need to drink your food and eat your water." As in, chew your food until it is liquefied, and don't gulp your water. Sip your drink. Chewing your food and sipping your water will help improve your digestion and help you feel more satisfied.

## Principle 4 Stay hydrated

Drink a glass of water and lemon juice as soon as you wake up in the morning. Keep a re-usable bottle of water at your desk. Drink one bottle before lunch and another bottle during the afternoon. Have a glass of water or herbal tea instead of indulging in sweets after dinner. At parties, hold and sip water from a glass so that your hands stay occupied and you don't become dehydrated.

## Principle 5 Avoid processed foods

Don't eat products if you can't pronounce their ingredients. Processed foods usually have limited nutritional value and contain tons of sugar, artificial sweeteners, and additives. Carry around a few unsalted nuts and an apple so that you never "have to" grab a candy bar.

Aim to eat nutritionally dense, fresh, unprocessed foods. When possible, cook at home so that you know exactly what is going into your food.

## Principle 6 Don't keep your food triggers in the house

What is the cost/benefit of tempting yourself? You may be disciplined tonight, and possibly even tomorrow, but eventually, you will give in. If you want a treat, go out and have a small portion at a restaurant or a friend's house.

# CHAPTER TAKE-AWAY

Contrary to most health and fitness media tag lines, adopting a healthier lifestyle is not just a matter of becoming dedicated or disciplined; the process of adopting a healthier lifestyle can't be divorced from one's emotions, stress levels, sleep patterns, genetics, self-confidence, resources, and current and past mental and physical health.

Be honest with yourself. Reflect on why you make your nutritional choices. Don't misrepresent reality — don't tell yourself you ate because you were hungry when really you were depressed. Figure out if you eat more when you are angry, sad, tired, or hurt. Don't tell yourself you had only two glasses of wine if you actually had four servings divided into two big glasses. The size of the glass counts! Don't tell yourself you had only one serving of dinner, when in reality you ate while cooking (this is classic me). Food counts even when it is not on your plate.

If you decide you want wine, enjoy the wine. Own and enjoy the choice you made. Then learn from the choice so that you can make a better choice next time. Or, if you decide to make the same unhealthy choice again, fine, you only live once. Just own the choice.

Always remember that your health quest is something you are doing for YOU!

Adopting a healthier lifestyle is about self-care. Care enough about yourself to put healthy food into your body. Eating fresh berries is a present to yourself, not a punishment. Deciding to eat processed crap full of preservatives is not a reward.

Gradually work to change your eating habits so that your taste buds evolve and you crave healthier foods.

It has taken me years, but I have managed to gradually make healthy eating my norm. Believe me, I was not born craving healthy foods. While I still love chocolate, I now see it as a special treat, not something for daily consumption. As for the triple-cheese pasta that I lived on as a teenager, I am now infinitely more satisfied by perfectly grilled chicken, a green salad with a sharp but light vinaigrette, and a pile of roasted fennel. At least 90 percent of the time, I don't have to stress over what choice to make. I naturally gravitate toward the healthier option.

Figure out the WWHH of your eating habits, and regardless of the diet you choose to follow, live by the Captain Obvious principles of health and wellness. Sure, drinking more water and being mindful of your portions might not seem flashy or innovative, but Captain Obvious suggestions are the cornerstones of long-term health.

No matter what diet or delivery system you are on, remember that moderation, mindfulness, fruits, vegetables, and a limited amount of processed foods are the foundation of healthy eating.

My habits and my tastes have evolved — so can yours. I know they can!

# CHAPTER 7

# ESTABLISH A HEALTH ENTOURAGE

Surround yourself with people who will help you succeed.

Clients often say (only half-jokingly, and mostly as a way to let themselves off the fitness hook) that they wish they were a celebrity, that celebrities have it easy. It is part of a celebrity's job to work out and stay fit, and having an entourage — full-time nutritionist, chef, assistant, and trainer — makes it almost impossible for them not to be fit.

My response is always a big smile and something like, "Absolutely, full-time help would make everything SO much easier, but if you think having an entourage would be useful, don't use not having one as an excuse. Create your own."

The important word here is *create*. Remember my advice from chapter 1, that adopting a healthier lifestyle is an active process. Create opportunities to be active and successful — form solutions rather than find reasons to abandon your goals.

Sure, there is obviously a kernel of truth to the "celebrities have it easy" lament; they are highly motivated to stay fit since their livelihood depends in part on maintaining a certain image, and having a trainer and a chef does take much of the planning, thought, and preparation out of adopting a healthy lifestyle.

BUT ... there are also many celebrities who struggle with their health. Having money and time doesn't automatically make you fit. Money can also buy drugs, alcohol, and copious amounts of unhealthy food. You have to choose to prioritize your health and choose to find opportunities to be active. Life is about creating solutions.

This next part may sound like a non sequitur, but bear with me.

Growing up, if I started to whine, my mom would say, "Kathleen, stop whining and finish this sentence. 'There is always a ...'"

I would then answer, "Solution."

My mom would then say, "Okay, then let's work on finding it."

When it comes to the "If I were a celebrity and it was part of my job to be fit, losing weight would be easy" lament, the trick is to focus on what celebrities are doing that you CAN reproduce, not what you CAN'T reproduce. Or, in other words — to paraphrase my mom — to find a solution.

Learn from fit people. Look for opportunities to be active. Look for solutions!

Stop using what other people have, and your envy of their experiences, as a reason to abandon your goals.

Cherry-pick the things that fit people and celebrities do that you can actually reproduce. Learn from their success. Be creative!

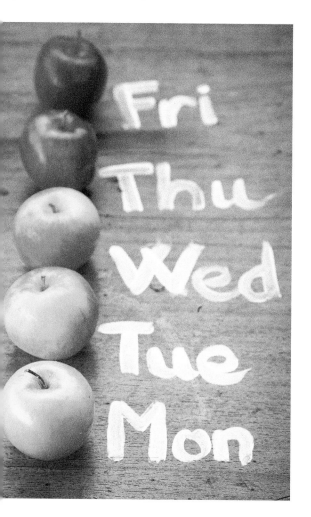

Improved health doesn't just happen. You have to actively set yourself up for health success. The more ways, the better!

# What Can You Learn from Celebrities?

· · · · · · · · · · · · · · · · · · · · · · · · · · · · · · · · · · · · · · · · · · · · · · · · · · · · · ·

What exactly is a health entourage, and how do you create one?

Basically, setting up a health entourage entails surrounding yourself with people who will help you succeed.

Celebrities maintain an active lifestyle for two main reasons, both of which you can reproduce (at least in part).

**Reason 1**   They are highly motivated to be healthy; often, their livelihood depends on being fit. So their desire to be healthy is driven by a strong WHY, or reason to be committed.

Find your unique health WHY — your inner motivation. Sure, you are not getting paid to be on the cover of a magazine, but there are lots of other good reasons why you should exercise. For example, decide you will strength train so that you will be strong enough to play with your grandkids, or take aquafit classes to decrease the pain of arthritis. For a more detailed explanation of how to find your WHY, refer back to chapter 1.

**Reason 2**   Celebrities stay fit because they have an entourage of health professionals. If you think having an entourage would be helpful, develop your own network of support. Many of your friends and family members are probably also struggling to adopt a healthier lifestyle, so connect with them. Establishing a health entourage is a great way to set yourself up for health success.

## Potential Members of Your Health Entourage (abbreviated version)

**1.** Supportive friends and family: These are people who are part of your health dream, but not in any tangible or physical way. They can simply be people who are encouraging of your process and thus provide moral support.

**2.** A gym or fitness buddy: Meet and work out with a friend, partner, spouse, colleague, or family member. Having someone to meet with will make you more accountable and will add a social element to the workout.

**3.** An accountability buddy: An accountability buddy does exactly what the name suggests. He or she makes you accountable to someone other than yourself, but you don't actually meet and train with them. I recommend accountability buddies to people who don't like the idea of training with someone or who can't realistically meet someone else because of scheduling or location issues. Email or call each other regularly to discuss anything and everything health related.

**4.** A nutrition buddy: Use your buddy simply as a nutritional sounding board. Discuss healthy recipes and healthy-eating strategies. Or, have a more hands-on buddy. Once a month, make a date with your buddy to cook together. Make six or eight healthy meals. Split the spoils and freeze for later.

**5.** Fitness or health groups or clubs: Join an already established club or create your own.

# Potential Members of Your Health Entourage (detailed version)

. . . . . . . . . . . . . . . . . . . . . . . . . . . . . . . . . . . . . . . . . . . . . . . . . .

## 1 Supportive friends and family

These members don't need to actually work out with you, or cook for you, or help you in any tangible or physical way. They can simply be people who are encouraging and provide moral support. They ask suitable questions, provide positive feedback, and offer a shoulder to cry on and an ear when needed. They absolutely shouldn't be people who try to sabotage your progress in any way. Get rid of anyone who urges you to have cake or drink wine when you are trying to abstain.

## 2 A fitness or gym buddy

This member of your entourage is fairly self-explanatory. Fitness buddies meet and work out together. You are less likely to skip your workout if you have someone waiting for you. Plus, a fitness buddy can make working out more fun.

Your fitness buddy can be a friend you meet at the gym, or your partner or spouse. Having a partner or spouse

who doubles as a fitness buddy can be a time-efficient way of nurturing your relationship. Stay active and connected at the same time; commit to doing fun activities on weekends, going on active holidays, and/or walking daily. I know many husband-and-wife couples who have set up a home gym so they can work out together in the evenings. I also train a number of husband-and-wife teams. If you can afford it, consider sharing a personal training session with your buddy.

Your buddy can even be your parent or child. I have mother-daughter teams who love training together. I myself enjoy going to yoga classes with my mom and then getting a coffee after. Having a fitness date is a nice excuse to be active and it ensures we see each other. Plus, my mom likes yoga and Zumba. I wouldn't usually try these types of classes, so training with her gives me variety and forces me to stretch. (I am terrible at making myself stretch. When I finish a run or a bike ride I want to shower and eat as quickly as possible. I too often sacrifice stretching. Doing yoga with my mom makes me dedicate an hour to improving my flexibility, which is important.) If

I challenge you — preferably you and a friend — to complete one "exercise adventure" each week for a month. Trying something new will breathe life into your routine and help break your fitness plateau. Plus, working out with a friend will help you stay accountable and will make the workout more fun. The adventure doesn't have to be big. It can be as simple as trying a new exercise or even a new variation on an exercise you already do. For example, if you always do stationary lunges, try walking lunges. Or pick a new running route, go to a new exercise class, or do a few extra repetitions of an exercise you already do. The adventure doesn't even have to take place during a gym workout; try a new sport or go on an active date with your significant other.

you don't want your buddy to be a family member, friend, or spouse, partner with a colleague at work; commit to walking or running at work on your lunch break. If your office has a gym, make a date with a friend to meet before, during, or after work. You are more likely to stop typing or get off the phone if you have someone waiting for you.

Just remember the Kathleenism from chapter 3: some movement is always better than no movement. Your health is like drops in a bucket. Every time you move, you accumulate health drops in your bucket. You might not think walking with a colleague for fifteen minutes a day or doing body-weight exercises in the living room with your partner will make a difference, but small choices, like drops, accumulate over time. Making regular dates with a buddy is a fantastic and fun way to accumulate your drops.

One note of caution — a buddy can be motivating, but she or he has to be the RIGHT buddy. Don't pick someone who will encourage you to ditch your workout at the slightest obstacle, and DON'T transfer the responsibility of training onto your partner.

Sure, a buddy can help keep you motivated, but the operative word is help. You still have to find the inner motivation to train. Your health process is exactly that: YOUR health process. When your buddy can't make a workout, that is not an excuse to skip your session. You have to commit to training regardless of what your buddy decides to do.

Frame your buddy as an added incentive, not as your driving force!

Remember what I said in chapter 2: Be your own health boss — stay in your own lane!

As a triathlete, I spend a lot of time running, cycling, and swimming, usually alone. When I first started competing, I loved being alone, in my zone, and always cycling, swimming, or running. In the winter of 2014, training started to feel a little like a chore. I am sure everyone reading can relate — I know that many people often find working out boring.

The thing is, I don't think exercise has to be, or should be, boring or tedious or a chore. Call me a fitness nerd, but I believe that movement has the potential to be empowering and enjoyable!

To help get myself out of my fitness rut, I decided I needed two things. I needed exercise to be more novel, and I needed to make exercise more social. So I enlisted my friend Jenn. Every Wednesday for a month we committed to trying a new exercise class — we called them Wedventures. We tried boxing class, Kangaroo Fitness, ballet barre, and Zumba. The variety did the trick. I had so much fun and I loved getting to see Jenn. Zumba put a smile on my face the ENTIRE time! We no longer have a Wedventure every week, but we try to participate in a new class at least once a month. We have tried interval rowing classes, TRX classes, spin, sandbag classes, and stand-up paddle boarding.

Wedventures taught me that having a fitness buddy is extremely motivating. I now know that going to fun fitness classes with a friend breathes new life into my routine, allows me to be social, and helps keep me accountable; I would never skip a workout if I know a friend is waiting. So whenever I feel myself getting into a fitness rut, I email a friend and make a date.

## 3 An accountability buddy

If working out with someone doesn't appeal to you, or isn't realistic based on your schedule or location, an alternative is to find an accountability buddy. An accountability buddy does exactly what the name suggests: he or she makes you accountable to someone other than yourself. You are more likely to get to that gym class or make a healthier food choice if you know you have to email or call your friend to debrief about your recent health choices. Decide to chat (either by email or phone) daily, weekly, or monthly. Make sure to schedule the times you will chat — if you don't decide when you will talk, life will simply take over. Good topics of conversation are your weekly exercise plans, your fitness goals, meal plans, possible roadblocks to success, and ideas for how to overcome those roadblocks.

I have a number of clients who have email accountability buddies. They commit to emailing at least once per week about their health struggles and successes. They discuss upcoming events that might be potential triggers, share recipes and websites, compare workouts, and generally offer a supportive ear.

## 4 A nutrition buddy

A nutrition buddy can help you in different ways. Nutrition buddies can be fairly hands-off.

### Hands-off buddy I: Nutritional sounding board

Your buddy can simply be a friend you use as a nutritional sounding board. Discuss healthy recipes and strategies for healthy eating together.

### Hands-off buddy 2: Cook and share

If you don't want to cook with your buddy, or your schedules don't permit you to meet, make food individually and split the spoils. That way you can have double the options of healthy food stored in your freezer. You will always have a quick and nutritious meal ready to go, and you will never have to reach for a frozen pizza.

Nutrition buddies can also be more hands-on.

### Hands-on buddy I: Cooking buddy

A cooking date is a great excuse to socialize, catch up, and prepare food for the month. Establish regular dates with your buddy; make six or eight healthy meals. There are tons of healthy soups and stews you can make in advance. Split the spoils and store the meals in your freezer. I have a number of mother-daughter pairs who meet regularly to make large quantities of four or five dishes. They each take home half to freeze, so that when they get home from work and need a quick meal, heating up something healthy will take just as long as warming up something unhealthy like a microwave pizza. The trick to healthy eating is preparation, preparation, preparation. When you make the process of preparing healthy options convenient and fun, you are more likely to maintain the habit long term.

### Hands-on buddy 2: Shopping buddy

You have to grocery shop anyway, so make it a social outing. Meet your buddy once a week at the grocery store or local farmers' market. Get lots of fresh local produce and catch up at the same time. As soon as you get home, cut up the produce and store it in containers so that when you're hungry after work, you have stuff to eat already cut up.

## 5 A fitness or health club

The more the merrier! Establish a fitness club — somewhat like a book club, but one that is centred on health. Meet once per month and discuss a health book or exchange health tips. Or decide to simply meet, chat, and offer other members a shoulder to lean on.

If you don't like the idea of a sedentary fitness club, create an active club that goes on weekly or monthly fitness adventures. Go running, organize a fitness adventure like rock climbing, go on active day trips to ski or snowshoe, try different fitness classes, or simply go for walks around the neighbourhood.

I had one group of clients who created a health group that was a really interesting mix of all three types of buddies. This particular client group discussed strategies for healthy eating and worked out together whenever they could. When their schedules didn't mesh, they emailed and checked in with one another instead.

Be creative — you can create any type of entourage your heart desires!

If you don't like the idea of creating a group, or you don't have friends who would be interested, join a pre-established one. For an active group, try the Running Room. The Running Room is a chain of stores that primarily sells running- and walking-related products — everything from athletic shoes to foam rollers. They also have weekly running groups. You can pay to join a group that is training for a particular event, or you can simply drop in on their community runs. Typically these community runs are Sunday mornings. If you are interested in finding an emotional support system, try Weight Watchers, or do some research online. The Internet is a wealth of information. If you are a new mom, find an active "mommy group" in your area. Many of my clients with babies find these groups extremely helpful. With a little creativity and perseverance, you will be amazed at what you can find.

Set your entourage up for success by establishing concrete, REALISTIC goals and a detailed action plan.

Setting up your entourage will not make you automatically fit. Don't just "wish" that you and your friend will meet up to work out or to cook — you have to follow through and actually exercise or get together and make food. You can't just talk; you have to actually DO.

Remember what I said in chapter 1: Adopting a healthier lifestyle is not a passive process; you have to actively set yourself up for health success. If you and your buddy both have busy lives, you will never actually meet unless you establish realistic goals and take the time to outline a detailed plan of attack.

I know I have said this before, but this point is key, so excuse my broken record: make sure your goals are realistic. Your goals need to reflect the realities of YOUR current life, not the realities of the life you used to have, or the life you want to have. If you just had a child or you have started a new job, your rhythms will be different. Make a plan of action based on your current responsibilities and financial reality. Your plan should include the WHAT, WHERE, WHEN, and HOW of your workout plan. (See chapter 4 for details.)

Never forget that it is not your health buddy's responsibility to make sure you train. He or she can be an added incentive, but ultimately, the buck stops with you. If your health buddy can't train, you still need to harness your inner WHY and make yourself move!

Remember what I said in chapter 4: Absent a concrete implementation plan, bold, sweeping health statements (or as I call them, fitness wishes) will most likely be forgotten as soon as life gets busy, which it inevitably does. Anticipate that and act accordingly. Don't just make statements like, "I will work out next week." That is more like a wish than a goal. The trick to making your fitness wishes come true is to establish realistic, safe, and sustainable long- and short-term goals.

First, look at everything in life as an opportunity to be active rather than as an excuse to be sedentary. Sure, you may be too busy to get to the gym, but you can always find ways to fit movement into your life. Second, don't try to change all your health habits at the same time. Establish a few realistic goals. Your first goal should be a "game changer" — the thing that will make the most impact on your overall health. Pick the unhealthy habit you do most often and start there. For example, if you drink pop, start by replacing pop with water. Make yourself accountable; write the goals down or tell them to your friends and family. Third, establish both long- and short-term goals. Breaking goals down into smaller, more manageable pieces can help you avoid feeling overwhelmed.

Last, don't set yourself up for failure. Set realistic goals that take into account your health history, current lifestyle, age, gender, and genetic makeup. Generalized weight-loss goals — like "I am going to lose twenty pounds" — are not useful. You might not need to lose twenty pounds. Maybe you need to lose five pounds of fat and gain muscle. Or maybe you have lost too much weight and need to gain weight. Everyone has a range of weight that is healthy to have on their frame, and we all feel better at different weights. I am six feet tall; just because another woman is six feet tall doesn't mean she will feel comfortable at my weight. Plus, I might feel comfortable at a different weight in twenty years than I do now. The amount

you need to lose is always relative to how much weight you have already lost, your height, your genetics, your age, and your exercise profile. Aim to be the best and healthiest version of yourself that you can be. Find a recipe for success that works for your individual body. Create your recipe by learning from past mistakes and by forming goals that are realistic and sustainable based on your lifestyle, and that are relevant and important to YOU. Tell your friends and family what you want to accomplish. Stating the goal out loud, so that other people know about your plans, can help keep you on track. In addition, write your goals down. Writing your goals down will help you be more accountable to yourself. Revisit this process every few months to assess your progress. If you have not been successful, brainstorm why. Then form new goals based on your new-found knowledge.

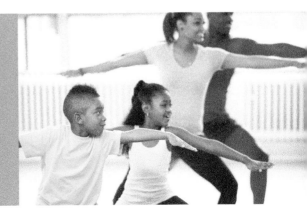

The more reasons you have to stick to your health quest, the better!

# CHAPTER TAKE-AWAY

Improving your health doesn't just happen — adopting a healthier lifestyle is an active process. The more healthy influences, positive triggers, and strategies you can establish for success, the better.

When you hit a roadblock — such as diminishing motivation — find a solution. A fantastic way to become more motivated (and to actively set yourself up for success) is to forge various health alliances. Establish an entourage of sorts — a network of people with common goals.

Your friends are your friends because they care about you and want you to succeed. You care about them and want them to succeed. So partner with them. Capitalize on your mutual desire for success — get yourself a fitness buddy, an accountability buddy, a nutrition buddy, or create a health group. Just remember, don't transfer the responsibility of your success onto your entourage. Don't think that if your buddy quits, you can quit, or that they will do the work for you. Ultimately, it is up to you to exercise and eat well.

Be prepared. Your partner will bail on you occasionally and you will be annoyed. Expect this. Instead of using your frustration as an excuse to skip your workout, harness your annoyance and use it as extra incentive to work out. Remember this Kathleenism: The worse your mood, the more important your workout. So, when you are unimpressed with your friend, work out to expel your frustration.

Last, remember that adopting a healthy lifestyle is not about discipline, it is about mindfulness and preparation. A large component of being prepared is identifying your triggers and solutions for them in advance.

Establish the entourage that fits your unique needs. If you know you are more likely to go to the gym with a friend, get a gym buddy. If you like working out alone but you can't get a handle on cooking healthy food, ignore my suggestion of a gym buddy and instead get yourself a nutrition buddy. Establish the entourage that will be the most helpful for YOU!

Look for opportunities to be active rather than reasons to be sedentary. Cherry-pick from other people's strategies; adopt what will work for you.

Find solutions! Create your unique recipe for health success.

When you have periods of low motivation, or your recipe for success isn't working for you, don't worry. We all fall off the fitness horse sometimes. The trick is to simply get back on a more informed rider. Learn from your less-than-ideal choices; frame them as opportunities for you to evolve and grow so that you can make better choices in the future.

# CHAPTER 8

# STOP FIXATING ON THE SCALE AND AIM TO GET OUT OF BODY DEBT

Don't conflate thinness with health. Becoming healthier is not just about the number on the scale. If your "health" regimen is making you feel worse about yourself, not better, rethink your plan. Adopting a healthier lifestyle should make you feel empowered and energized, not judged and deprived.

The "body debt/body credit" system refers to each individual's level of overall health. Body credit is your level of energy, vitality, and physical resilience. You accumulate credit by making healthy choices that help your body recover, such as sleeping enough, eating well, exercising appropriately, and stretching.

You deplete your credit by consciously or unconsciously making unhealthy choices such as sitting for hours, going on extreme diets, or eating unhealthfully.

Body debt occurs when the amount you ask of your body (for example, asking it to survive on processed foods or to sit for hours without a break) exceeds the amount of time and energy you put into recovery (like sleeping enough and eating healthy food).

Or, put another way, debt occurs when your unhealthy habits outnumber your healthy habits.

You are in debt if you are always tired, always injured, always cranky, have a hard time maintaining or losing weight, and have a hard time sleeping.

Unfortunately, yo-yo diets and extreme exercise routines deplete credit. Too many people exercise and watch their diet only when they want to lose weight, and they use the scale as their sole barometer of success. The almost inevitable result is yo-yo dieting and exercise patterns — vacillation between periods of extreme, unsustainable control and disregard for health. Sure, people don't always admit outright that they are trying to lose weight — they might say, "I am trying to get healthier" — but in my experience, in their heart of hearts, "get healthier" is code for "become thinner" or "look more like my favourite celebrity." They either consciously or unconsciously use "health" as a code word for dieting, losing weight, or looking a certain way. I get it — most of us (including myself) have a complicated relationship with our bodies; the lines between dieting, health, weight, and self-esteem often become blurred.

The thing is, in my experience, fixating on the scale doesn't help anyone make sustainable healthy changes or keep weight off in the long term; conflating health with reaching a certain weight is counterproductive.

Fixating on the scale does not amass credit! Too many people weigh themselves daily when in weight-loss mode. I am not a fan of daily weigh-ins; weighing yourself daily feeds into this yo-yo mentality and is not ultimately healthy or helpful. Plus, the idea that one should weigh in daily feeds into a discourse of weight loss and health that I find incredibly frustrating — the discourse that there is a quick fix to becoming healthier, and that "health" is actually just a synonym for "becoming thinner."

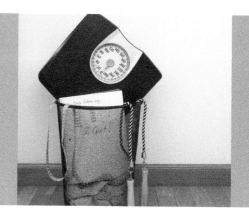

Remember, you can always find ways to be active if you look at everything in life as an opportunity.

In my experience, when people weigh themselves daily, they start basing how they feel about themselves on whether they have gained or lost weight on the scale. We are all more than a number; how we feel day to day should not depend on what we see on the scale.

Further, weekly or monthly weigh-ins are more accurate because they show real weight loss versus what I refer to as "fake weight." The 0.1 or 0.2 pounds you gain or lose day to day is not an indication of true fat loss. It is an indication of hydration levels, the amount of salty foods you ate the day before, and whether you went to the bathroom before getting on the scale.

I suggest that if you want to weigh in regularly, the most frequently you should do it is weekly, or at the most, twice weekly. Pick one or two days of the week and always weigh yourself on those days, at a particular time, wearing the same clothes (or lack thereof) each time.

We all fluctuate in weight by a few pounds. That is normal. If you want to lose weight, try not to worry about your daily minuscule fluctuations — fixating daily on a number can be demoralizing and counterproductive! Instead, your aim should be to fluctuate downward. If in January you fluctuate between 180 and 185, aim to fluctuate between 175 and 180 by February or March. your day-to-day fluctuations are less important than your weekly, monthly, or yearly trends. Don't get caught up in the trees — see the "forest." Think long-term — focus on trending positive.

Health (and the quest to amass credit) should not be understood as simply your weight on the scale. Health should be understood as an intersection of how you look, how you feel, your nutrition and exercise habits, your lifestyle, and your genetics.

Don't just try to reach a certain number on the scale. Instead, work toward getting out of body debt by establishing a plethora of HEALTH goals, including improved sleep, being stronger, and eating more fruits and vegetables.

I will explain the body debt/body credit system in more detail later in this chapter, but first let me explain why focusing on the number on the scale — and thinking that "thin" and "healthy" are the same thing — is ultimately not healthy or helpful.

# Three Reasons Why Fixating on the Scale is Ultimately NOT Helpful

. . . . . . . . . . . . . . . . . . . . . . . . . . . . . . . . . . . . . . . . . . . . . . . .

| Losing weight isn't always
the most useful health goal

Although losing weight would positively affect many people's health, others don't actually NEED to lose weight; they need to gain muscle or improve their cardiovascular health. Many people WANT to lose weight, but needing to lose weight for health reasons and wanting to lose weight for aesthetic reasons are two different things.

Obviously, I strongly believe that everyone should exercise, but "exercise" should not be synonymous with "weight loss." Some people are thin and weak. What they need is to gain muscle. Others may have already lost weight. To lose more might be unhealthy. Others, and this is common (I know I have succumbed to this), want to lose weight, but the weight loss is not a health objective. If I say I "need" to lose weight, what that means is "I don't feel my best athletically when I am five pounds heavier," or "I would like to feel more comfortable in a certain outfit." Perspective is key — when people are within their healthy weight range, needing to lose weight and wanting to lose weight are two different things.

There are a number of body-weight classification systems. The most accurate test to determine how much fat versus muscle you have is the dual-energy x-ray absorptiometry (DEXA) machine. It actually produces a body-fat map, which outlines exactly where your fat is distributed throughout your body. Unfortunately, it is expensive and not easily accessible. I have never even had it done.

Two common and accessible body-weight classification systems are the BMI (body mass index) and the waist/hip ratio test. BMI is calculated by dividing your weight in kilograms by the square of your height in metres. For example, if your weight is sixty kilograms and your height is 1.7 metres, your BMI is 21. The BMI assumes that there is no perfect weight for any one height, but rather a range of healthy weights. A healthy BMI is between 18.5 and 25. A BMI below 18.5 or above 25 puts one at a greater risk of acquiring certain health conditions, such as heart disease. For a quick online BMI calculator, visit www.whathealth.com.

Your waist/hip ratio helps to pinpoint how your fat is distributed on your body. This is helpful because the way our fat is distributed (not just our overall weight) impacts our health risk. Excess weight around your middle puts you at a greater risk of lifestyle-related diseases such as diabetes and heart disease. Your waist/hip ratio is your waist measurement (in inches or centimetres) divided by your hip measurement. First, measure the distance around the smallest area of your waist, usually just above the belly button. This will give you your waist circumference. Then, measure the distance around the largest area of your hips. This will give you your hip circumference. Women should have a ratio of 0.8 or less. Men should aim to have a ratio of 0.95 or less. A ratio of 1.0 or higher puts an individual in the "at risk" category for heart disease and other problems associated with being overweight.

If you are within your healthy weight range, don't confuse wanting to lose five pounds for aesthetic reasons with needing to lose weight for health reasons. Striving to be thin or perfectly toned can be the opposite of healthy. Fixation on your weight, especially if you are within your healthy zone, is not usually psychologically healthy and can lead to a compulsive relationship with food and exercise. Plus, for women especially, being too thin can have dramatic negative effects on health. If fat stores fall too low, hormonal imbalances and menstrual irregularities result.

Often, during the times in my life that I was at my smallest pant size, my relationship with my body was the least healthy, and I didn't like myself much. People complimented me on my weight, but I was physically and emotionally unhappy in my own skin. It may sound silly, but I hated when people complimented me on how I looked because it made me feel judged; I felt that if they noticed I had lost weight, then they must have noticed when I was heavier. The truth is that I spent that portion of my life constantly feeling judged; I didn't even really like working out or eating with people because I never felt like I could enjoy the experiences. I felt sort of like an animal at the zoo — always being watched. At that point in my health journey I couldn't do what I now tell my clients to do, which is to "stay in my own health lane." I now know that it doesn't matter what others think about what I eat, my exercise routine, or how I look. All that matters is that I am making decisions that the future Kathleen will be proud of, decisions that will help me grow into the healthy, happy, and well-balanced Kathleen that I am continually working to become. The only criteria that matter for who this happy and healthy Kathleen will be are mine. I have to stay in my lane, just as my friends and family have to stay in theirs.

Striving for a particular aesthetic can be a manifestation of obsessive control, wrapped in the facade of becoming healthier.

I am not saying that if you are within your healthy range you should never want to lose five pounds, I am just saying, don't lie to yourself and pretend it is about your health. OWN that it is an aesthetic choice. (Owning health choices is always paramount.)

## 2 Losing weight in an unhealthy way — even when weight loss is needed — is not beneficial to your long-term physical or psychological health

In my experience, people too often resort to unhealthy tactics when they fixate on the scale — think calorie-restrictive diets and intense workout sessions. Not only do restrictive diets and unrealistic workout programs foster body hate, they also don't give the body the nutrients it needs to thrive. Overworking the body — especially while also undernourishing it — puts the body at risk of injury, malnourishment, exhaustion, and hormone irregularity, all of which are disincentives to train.

If you feel like crap — because you are exhausted from malnourishment or injured from overtraining — you are more likely to fall off the fitness horse, which ultimately means you won't achieve your weight-loss goal anyway. Thus, fixating on the scale is not only potentially physically and psychologically damaging, it is also counterproductive.

## 3 Making weight loss your number-one objective sets you up for long-term failure

If you exercise only when you are on a diet and trying to lose weight, you end up associating movement with being in weight-loss mode.

Consciously or unconsciously conflating health with thinness fosters an unhealthy relationship with your body, food, and exercise. The almost inevitable result is yo-yo dieting and exercise patterns — vacillation between unhealthy, extreme dieting and binge eating between periods of overtraining and sedentary behaviour.

Make movement a non-negotiable, something you just always do, not something you do only when you are trying to look good for a wedding.

If you exercise only to look a certain way, and exercising doesn't result in the look you are working toward, you will feel discouraged and have a strong disincentive to move.

The more varied your goals, the more likely you will be to continue to move, regardless of how exercise is making you look.

Don't get caught up in reaching a certain weight and in the process take your body for granted. Becoming healthier is not just about the number on the scale. Working out should make you feel more energized and empowered, not judged or defeated. When you don't want to work out, or if you become discouraged when the scale won't budge, think big picture. Remind yourself that movement is a privilege and that the point of moving is not solely to lose weight — it is to feel stronger, to have more energy, and to improve your overall health.

Who wants to continue doing something they don't like, especially when they aren't getting the desired result?

One can't control exactly how the body will react to exercise; every individual, depending on their age, gender, exercise history, and genetics will respond to exercise differently. I will never look like Serena Williams or win an Olympic marathon. Two women might both be able to get down to 110 pounds, but the first might be able to do so and still have occasional treats. The second might have to deprive herself of everything, and may even lose her period, to maintain that weight. The second woman may be happier, and ultimately healthier, five or ten pounds heavier.

I am not advocating that you use genetics as an excuse for unhealthy behaviour. Genetics predispose you to react to food, exercise, and your environment in a certain way, but it does not produce a finite conclusion.

What I am saying is that moving is always healthy, regardless of how it makes

your body look. So establish multiple goals, like having more energy and drinking more water. Varied goals will encourage you to exercise, regardless of how exercise is making you look.

Moving is always healthy, whether or not you are trying to lose weight.

I am not arguing that weight loss shouldn't be one of your goals, just don't use losing weight as your only barometer of health success.

Frame your health process as a quest to amass body credit and get out of body debt — if you have excess weight to lose, consider losing it as simply one way to accumulate credit.

The more reasons you have to stay on your fitness horse, the more likely you are to actually get yourself out of body debt and amass body credit. The more credit you develop, the healthier you will be.

So instead of fixating on the number on the scale, aim to accumulate body credit and get out of body debt!

# The Body Debt/Body Credit System

To recap, body credit is a concept I use to explain each individual's level of overall health — their body's unique ability to resist physical stress. Basically, it is the body's level of energy, vitality, and physical resilience.

Everyone's body credit fluctuates throughout their life. Age and genetics predispose people to a certain level of credit and help to determine how quickly one's credit replenishes itself, but everyone should always be working to accumulate credit. It is ALWAYS possible to accumulate credit; you are either accumulating credit or accumulating debt.

## Activities that Accumulate Debt

Unhealthy habits such as eating to excess, being overweight, being inactive, not sleeping enough, having poor posture, sitting too much, eating too many preservatives, and drinking too many sugary drinks instead of water all incur debt.

Debt can also be accumulated by exercising too intensely and not recovering appropriately. When you push your body and don't recover at an appropriate rate, you go into body debt. As an athlete I have to be very careful not to go into debt. Overtraining is very dangerous. It is easy to

start buying into the training concept that more is always better, but as I tell my clients, "More is not better; better is better."

When you exercise intensely, especially when you do it sporadically and your body is not used to it, you risk incurring massive amounts of debt.

Sedentary lifestyles use up as much or more body credit as active lifestyles do.

Being inactive is bad for your long-term cardiovascular health, and sitting is hard on your entire musculoskeletal system. This is especially true if you are sitting with bad posture, which, let's face it, most of us are. Bad posture taxes our structural system and therefore uses more credit, causing muscles to get stiff and sore.

Unhealthy habits — such as being sedentary or eating a high-sugar diet — will

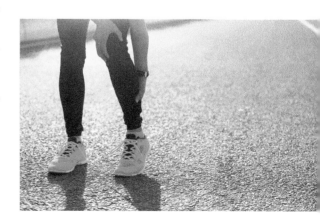

decrease your credit. If your credit decreases enough, the result is body debt.

Debt occurs when you chronically make unhealthy choices. A good goal is to make more daily healthy choices than unhealthy ones. Now, I am not saying you can't have a few less-healthy habits. We all need a beer (or in my case, a few chocolate almonds) once in a while, but you have to be mindful of your less-than-stellar choices so that the rest of your choices can be healthier, and you mitigate the damages of a less-healthy choice with a healthier one. When you are not aware of your detrimental choices — or, as I say to clients, "When you make multiple willy-nilly unhealthy choices" — you put yourself at risk of going into (or further into) debt.

Sure, some of us pretend to take care of ourselves — we stretch for five minutes after a run or get up once every four hours from our computer to walk around — but most of us don't really take recovery and making healthy choices seriously. We diet and exercise sporadically, usually in an unhealthy way, and the rest of the time we ask way more of our bodies than is possible. We deplete our bodies' energy stores and go into debt.

It is no wonder that so many of us consistently feel slightly stiff, achy, tired, lethargic, or tight. Most of us make willy-nilly unhealthy choices — we have used up all of our body credit and gone into debt.

## Activities that Amass Credit

Stretching, eating well, sleeping, allowing for appropriate recovery between workouts, staying hydrated, and being appropriately active all amass credit.

Getting out of body debt is not a one-time quick fix. You can't stretch for a week or go to physio once and think you will have repaid your body debt. Repaying

I know from personal experience that building back one's credit is a long, hard process. In 2014 I injured my left calf. Training for an Ironman and a marathon had overtaxed my system; I was in body debt. After my marathon I thought I could take a couple weeks off and magically I would be okay. That was like saying ten dollars could pay off a million-dollar debt. I put my body through hell for eight months. Ten days was not enough recovery. It took me almost a year to feel like my old self again.

your debt will take hard, continuous effort, especially if you have been using up your body's credit for years.

If you have aches and pains, don't feel discouraged if you don't improve quickly. A sore shoulder or hip due to bad posture or a faulty gait can take years to materialize. Don't be fooled. Yes, there may have been a moment when you finally felt the pain, but your body debt has most likely been building for years.

The more debt you have and the older you are, the longer it will take you to amass credit and the harder you will have to work to get out of debt.

So many of us continually drain our bodies' resources without proportionally repaying our debt. Unfortunately, as we age, it gets easier to go into debt and takes much more work to replenish the bank!

If you sit a lot, you need to work hard to replenish your body's bank. If you have been sitting with bad posture for years, a few haphazard neck stretches will not get rid of your neck pain.

. . . . . . . . . . . . . . . . . . . . . . . . . . .

Remember what I said in chapter 4: Don't just make a fitness wish. If you actually want to get out of debt, you need to take the time to figure out a plan of attack. Here are a few "get out of debt" action plans.

If you have incurred debt from ...

## Lack of sleep

Don't state something akin to a wish, such as "I will sleep more." Take the time to figure out HOW you will sleep more. If you have trouble falling asleep, maybe you need to create a bedtime ritual. Turn off all screens thirty minutes before bed. Meditate, journal, or do some deep breathing. Follow the same routine each night so that you train your body to get used to sleeping.

## Eating fast food

Aim to make more of your food at home, but don't just say, "I won't eat fast food." Instead, plan in advance how you will make healthy food. Decide in advance what meals you will make for dinner and make extra so that you can bring leftovers to work for your lunch.

## Sitting too much

Set an hourly alarm. When the alarm goes off, get up and walk around and do a minimum of one stretch. If possible, get an ergonomic assessment of your workspace, and take as many of your telephone meetings as possible while walking.

One way to get out of debt is to recover like an athlete. Athletes train hard, but they also recover well. They have to recover because, although working out is healthy, it stresses the body and causes tissue breakdown. Since muscles repair and get stronger during recovery, smart athletes focus on proper

Appreciate that you can be active and exercise, and that you have access to healthy food, versus fixating on the things that you perceive you are denying yourself. For example, I often want to keep sleeping when my alarm goes off. To convince myself to get out of bed and get on my bike, I remind myself that I am lucky to have a racing bike and to be healthy enough to be able to ride it, and that training will make me feel great. I focus on the positive aspects of training rather than dwelling on the negative fact that cycling will mean I can't sleep in.

post-workout nutrition, proper hydration, stretching, getting massages, and sleeping.

How you treat your body when you are not training is just as important as what you do to your body during training. In my opinion, recovery is the most undervalued training variable. Recovery can help you feel stronger, more agile, and less achy.

Remember, the amount of time you need to put into your recovery has to be proportional to the amount of debt you are in. Part of getting out of debt is being realistic about what your body can do by setting realistic goals. Respect your body's "window" and work to maximize your potential. Don't ask something of your body that is not possible. I had to come to terms with this myself. There was a time in my life I wanted to finish a marathon in 3:00 to 3:30 hours. Then I realized that if I tried, I would hurt myself. For me, aiming for a 3:40 marathon would be a challenge, but an appropriate one. I don't have the genetics to be a world-class runner — and that is okay. I can be the best runner I can be.

To quote my dad, my goal is always to take my genetics and hit a home run. Now, as I tell my clients, you can hit this metaphorical home run by how you exercise and eat, as well as by how you frame your life experiences.

Hit a mental home run by being positive and not comparing yourself to others. Constantly comparing and criticizing your body usually causes frustration, anxiety, or guilt. These emotions can produce the opposite end result than intended.

Don't stay away from the gym until you become more fit just because you don't want people witnessing how unfit you are. Talk about a self-fulfilling prophecy! You won't become more fit unless you move.

Find the positive in the fact that you can move, versus fixating on the friend you don't look like or the body shape you realistically won't create.

Having negative thoughts about your body is another way to accumulate body debt; negative thoughts don't help you become a more vital and energetic human being. Stop comparing yourself to other people or to an ideal version of yourself. Just move.

# CHAPTER TAKE-AWAY

Set yourself up for health success, and stop fixating on the scale.

Aim to get out of body debt by having more healthy habits than unhealthy habits; establish realistic, specific, and measurable goals. Focus on becoming stronger and fitter, not just on weighing less. Reframe how you understand "adopting a healthier lifestyle." Instead of understanding health as synonymous with weight, and associating being "healthier" with deprivation and austerity, understand eating well and exercising more as a way to feel stronger and more powerful, to have more energy, and to improve your overall health. Working out should make you feel energized and empowered, not deprived and frustrated.

Care about fat loss, not just about the number on the scale! If you do need to lose weight, determine what your healthy weight range would be based on your height, age, gender, and fitness history. Remember that we all fluctuate in weight by a few pounds. When trying to lose weight, your aim should be to fluctuate downward.

If you do need to lose weight, think of losing weight as playing the stock market. The day-to-day fluctuations are less important than the weekly, monthly, or yearly trends. Weighing in daily and obsessing about the small numbers is like focusing on a grain of sand and ignoring the beach.

The benefits of exercise extend far beyond weight loss. The positive effects of exercise include improved sleep, energy, mood, long-term health, mobility, strength, and athletic achievement. Try to establish health, wellness, and athletic goals — not just aesthetic goals — based on these factors. If your goals are not making you feel positive about yourself, maybe you need to rethink them. Maybe you are asking something of your body that is not genetically possible.

Move away from short-term, unrealistic health resolutions. Instead, aim to amass credit so that you get out of debt. The more debt you are in, the harder it will be to start moving and adopt a healthier lifestyle. Getting out of body debt will help you have the energy and vitality to stay injury-free and motivated to move long term. Make small, realistic changes that you can maintain for the rest of your life. Try to stop judging the bodies of yourself and others. Instead, use that energy to get up and go for a walk or to reflect on your own relationship with your body and not on what your body looks like that day. Health is a process — our habits, emotions, and level of fitness develop gradually over time in overlapping and intertwining layers.

# CHAPTER 9

# WAYS YOU MIGHT BE UNKNOWINGLY SABOTAGING YOUR PROGRESS

People who have successfully changed their lifestyle succeeded because they persevered. I didn't become a healthier version of myself overnight. I adopted the mindset that "health" is not a finite goal: I am dedicated to making every day a learning experience. When I fall off my health horse, I get back on immediately and make sure I'm a more informed rider. Health is a lifelong process — and a non-linear one. It takes daily dedication, self-reflection, and long-term goal setting.

It just plain sucks to give it your all and still not reach your health goals. It is one thing not to reach your health and wellness goals if you are eating fries every day and skipping workouts, but it is extremely frustrating to work hard and still not succeed. Believe me, I get it. I have broken down in tears from not getting the personal best I thought I deserved after training for months.

If you feel you are doing everything right but are still not accomplishing your health goals, you may be unknowingly sabotaging your own progress. Keep reading. This chapter is for you.

In my experience, most people who aren't reaching their health goals are making one of the following four health missteps: they don't strength train, they get inadequate recovery, and they ignore the importance of either high-intensity interval workouts or of being mindful.

To figure out if you are making one of these four mistakes, journal your exercise, eating, sleeping, and drinking habits for two weeks. Note anything that may be important. This data will help you decipher if you are making (unintentionally or intentionally) one of these health missteps. Journaling is imperative, since most of us overestimate the healthy choices we make and underestimate the unhealthy choices we make. (For a detailed description of how to keep a journal, refer to chapter 6.)

When you analyze the data from your journal, take a moment to reflect on whether your goals are realistic. Your lack of success might be simple — you might be asking your body to do something that is not possible or healthy. Or, you might be expecting a miracle from your schedule. If you work fourteen hours a day don't aim to go to the gym daily for two hours — that is just setting yourself up to fail. You either have to change your work schedule or form more realistic goals. Or you might have too many competing goals. Don't try to change all your health habits at once. Prioritize — decide which changes will give you the

The feeling of being alone in "the struggle" can be demoralizing, so try to keep in mind that health is a daily learning process, even for people who seemingly have it all figured out. Making healthier choices is never easy; making healthier choices simply becomes easier. Take me. I love Fudgsicles. The process of learning how to healthfully indulge in fudge bars (because I don't believe that complete deprivation is healthy either) has been complicated. Now, obviously one fudge bar is fine. The problem is that I know myself, and if I buy a box I will consume the whole thing — even though I tell myself I will eat only one bar every few days. The first few times I made the goal of "no more fudge" were utterly disastrous. I would hit the frozen-food aisle and the devil on my shoulder would say, "You can be disciplined. You can have Fudgsicles in the freezer and eat only one." I learned (after many tries) that I can't. So, it is now a non-negotiable — I don't keep a box in the house. When I want a fudge bar, I buy a single bar from the convenience store. The best part is that by eating one bar (not six) I always enjoy it and don't feel guilty. I have learned that the second (and third) bar never tastes as good as the first.

most bang for your buck, then start there. For example, if you eat well during the day and then pig out after 10 p.m., don't waste your energy changing your meals. Decide to stop snacking after dinner, or at least decide on healthier parameters for your snacking. Basically, you need a detailed and realistic plan of action; your goals need to reflect how much time and energy you actually have (not how much you want to have), your finances, and your equipment. Fitness wishes — without corresponding action — will never come true.

You may find that once you form fewer, more realistic goals, you start to (almost magically) be successful.

Step 1    Stop using the "I am too busy" excuse. Even if you are too busy to get to the gym, you can ALWAYS find ways to be active if you look at everything in life as an opportunity for activity.

Step 2    Don't aim to change all your health habits at once. Establish two or three realistic goals. Make a plan of action. Figure out in advance the WHAT, WHERE, WHEN, and HOW of your workout plan.

Step 3    Establish both long-term and short-term goals. Break your goals down into smaller, more manageable pieces to avoid feeling overwhelmed.

Step 4    Set specific, individually tailored goals. Don't set yourself up for failure — make realistic goals that take into account your health history, current lifestyle, age, gender, and genetic makeup.

Step 5    No two individuals react to an exercise regimen in the same way — everyone's fitness and health journey will be unique. Learn from your past mistakes and form goals that are realistic and sustainable based on your lifestyle, and that are relevant and important to YOU.

For a more detailed description of how to make goals, not wishes, refer to chapter 4. But for now, here's how you can start.

Once you have made sure your goals are realistic, analyze the data in your journal. Ask yourself if you are making one (or more) of the following common health missteps.

# Four Common Health Missteps

. . . . . . . . . . . . . . . . . . . . . . . . . . . . . . . . . . . . . . . . . . . . . . . . . . .

## Misstep 1 — Not strength training

Too many people prioritize cardiovascular exercise (like running) over strength training. One of my favourite Kathleenisms is, don't do cardio to get into shape; get into shape to do cardio. Cardio — especially high-impact cardio such as running — is hard on the body. Prioritizing cardio can be detrimental to the body over the long term. Strength training makes you strong enough to do cardio, strengthens your bones to help prevent osteoporosis, and ensures that you are strong enough to withstand life's challenges.

In fact, the more you love cardio, and the more you use cardio as a method of weight control, the more important strength and balance work become, because if you get injured, it will be harder for you to do cardio. The inability to stand on one leg for ten seconds (balance) or perform a squat (strength) have both been shown to be strong indicators of future injuries and even mortality. I don't want to be injured — running always puts me in a better mood. I can't imagine how unhappy I would be if I couldn't run. My love of running incentivizes me to strength train — to

do exercises such as squats and single-leg balance exercises. The main take-away thus far? Strength train!

Need more incentive to strength train? Are you doing hours of cardio in an attempt to change your physique or lose weight? Strength training will help transform your body's shape. Plus, strength training helps increase your metabolism. Now, a clarification. When I say "strength training," I am not talking about core work. Most people I know who hate strength training love a good core session. By "strength training" I mean exercises like squats, lunges, deadlifts, and push-ups.

Learn from my mistakes. I resisted fully embracing strength training for a long time. I have always done weights, but I never prioritized them as highly as my triathlon training, and I always lifted light to moderate weights for twelve to fifteen reps. I emphasized my running and cycling over strength training, which led to overuse injuries and slower race times. Learning to incorporate strength and balance training has made me a stronger and less injury-prone athlete. I am proud to admit that I now enjoy my strength sessions (which include flipping tires and strength exercises like deadlifts) as much

Attention, every woman reading this — don't be afraid to strength train! Almost once per day a woman says to me, "I don't lift weights because I don't want to get too bulky."

It is 2016! Being strong is not a bad thing! Being strong is awesome; being strong will help you do everyday activities with ease, prevent injuries, promote proper posture, and strengthen your bones. Strength exercises, and the muscles that come with them, are a good thing. For me, strong legs allow me to attack hills while running and to cycle with ease, and a strong upper body helps me pull myself through the water during triathlons with power and precision.

Plus, it is almost impossible for a woman to get big, bulky muscles unless she REALLY tries — it is just not in our genetics. Unless an individual is predisposed to gaining muscle, bulking up takes dedication and a concentrated effort to consume enough calories. Do you know how hard most men have to work to get the muscle bulk they desire? Your thirty minutes of squats and lunges is not going to make you the Hulk. Even many men who do prioritize strength training still find that it takes dedication to elicit a hypertrophic (muscle growth) response.

You need to eat enough food to build muscle. Most women are too concerned with dieting and low-calorie foods to ever eat enough to gain significant muscle. Plus, in general, to create a hypertrophic response you need to do four-plus sets of an exercise with an appropriately heavy weight for six to twelve repetitions. Most women don't lift within that range, and if they do, they don't use a weight heavy enough to lead to hypertrophy. If you do ten reps of an exercise with a weight you could actually manage twenty reps with (as many woman do), hypertrophy will not occur.

as most of my runs. For an endurance junkie like me, that is BIG. I'm hopeful that I learned my lesson early enough that future Kathleen doesn't have to have a double hip replacement.

To avoid constantly being derailed by injury, I prioritize multi-joint functional exercises such as squats, as well as single-leg balance exercises. To increase your overall metabolism, prioritize all multi-joint exercises such as push-ups, pull-ups, bent-over rows, squats, deadlifts, and lunges. As you get stronger, challenge yourself to lift heavier weights.

Main take-away: Strength train to improve your metabolism, to change the shape of your body, and to ensure that you are functionally strong. If you are a cardio junkie (I get it — I am a recovering one), and you use cardio as a mood booster or a way to keep your weight in check, make yourself strength train. Cardio — especially high-intensity or endurance cardio — is hard on the body. It can wreak havoc on your connective tissue, bones, and immune system. It can also mess with your hormones. Resistance and balance exercises will help you stay injury-free (or at least injury-light), meaning that you will be able to continue your love affair with cardio for life.

# Misstep 2  Lack of Recovery

By "recovery," I don't mean sitting on your sofa and eating chips while you watch TV.

By "recovery," I mean consciously giving your body the tools it needs to prosper. Recovery techniques include stretching, sleeping, eating well, getting regular massages or learning self-massage techniques, and doing active recovery motions such as walking or swimming.

Recovery can also be understood as anything that increases body credit. For a detailed explanation of the body debt/body credit system, refer to chapter 8. The body debt/body credit system refers to a person's level of overall health. Body credit is the pep in your step and your ability to recover and bounce back from stressful life experiences (for example, long days of work or intense workouts). Basically, "credit" is

## BENT-OVER ROW

→ Start standing, holding a dumbbell in each hand. Draw your shoulders back and engage your core. Hinge forward at your hips. Make sure you don't round through your upper back — keep your back flat, chest out, and shoulders back. Your arms should be straight, the dumbbells hanging toward the floor. This is your starting position.

→ Pull your elbows up toward the ceiling until your hands are on either side of your chest. Use your upper back, not your biceps to do the work. Hold for a second and then slowly release. Repeat for ten to fifteen repetitions.

energy and resilience. I know I am lacking in credit when it takes me until Thursday to recover from an intense day of training on Sunday; my inability to recovery indicates that my physical resilience is low.

Another way to think of the "debt/credit" system is with what I refer to as the "energy pie." Imagine this: We all wake up every day with a hundred pieces of pie. When you are in body debt, something that commonly would take you one piece of pie (like getting out of bed), might take you ten pieces of pie. When I am in debt, a long Sunday workout will take me thirty pieces of pie versus five. The end result of everything taking more pieces of pie is that you feel lethargic and energy depleted; by three o'clock all of your pie has been used up and you want to go to bed.

You accumulate credit (or resilience and pep) by making healthy choices that help your body recover, such as sleeping, eating well, exercising appropriately, and stretching. You deplete your credit by consciously or unconsciously making unhealthy choices such as sitting for hours, going on extreme diets, or eating unhealthfully. Body debt occurs when your unhealthy habits outnumber your healthy habits.

Exercise (especially high-impact activities like running) stresses the body. Exercise is a positive stress only if you give your body the ingredients it needs to recover; exercise helps your body get stronger only if you give it adequate time to recover. Training too intensely for too long can result in overuse injuries. On the other end of the spectrum, inadequate movement also stresses the body. If you are asking your body to sit for hours on end, you also have to give your body the tools it needs to recover from being forced into a sustained negative posture for so long.

Recovery is not just something you fit in if you have time.

Prioritize getting seven or more hours of sleep each night. Your body recovers while you sleep.

Be mindful of your nutrition. A healthy diet helps your muscles and connective tissue repair and become stronger.

Schedule time to stretch, and get regular body work like massage, or use a foam roller. The more you use your body, the more it requires regular body work.

Too much training and too little recovery is a recipe for injury. Learn to listen to your body. Don't push through aches and pains. That doesn't mean I think you should skip your workout and lie on your sofa. If your body needs a break from high-intensity activities, find other ways to be active. Try water running, where you run on the bottom of the pool in the shallow end or simulate the motion of running in the deep end, or take a Pilates class.

Copy me: multitask. Stretch and use a foam roller, a HyperIce Vyper roller, or yoga tune-up balls while you watch TV. The HyperIce Vyper is a roller that vibrates, thus offering a more intense massage. Yoga tune-up balls are small balls that you can use to release your entire body. Think of a tennis ball with slightly less give. Tune-up balls offer a more targeted release than a foam roller. Tell yourself you can watch TV only if you are stretching or using a roller for the first fifteen minutes.

For the past four Februarys I have taken the month off from running. Not running is brutally hard for me, but I figure if I have to give up my passion, I should do it in the winter. I hate being cold!

I always hate the first few days of the challenge — running is my bliss — but I want to run for the rest of my life, so I have to treat my body with respect.

I always survive the month. In large part that's because after about three days I remember how much I love trying different fun fitness classes and getting to row more. I rowed in high school and still love it. Rowing gives me the same full-body, athletic, intense workout as running, without the impact.

The main take-away is that part of recovering is experimenting. Let your body heal with variety. If you always bike, try running. If you always run, try rowing. Who knows, you might find another form of exercise you enjoy. The more varieties of exercise you like, the more likely you are to stay active. One of the reasons I am active is that most of the time I don't have to force myself to run. I want to run; it makes me happy. So experiment and find things you enjoy. If you like dogs, walk your dog. Or perhaps try a new sport.

Remember that you are only ever one workout away from a better mood. Find lots of ways to be active so that you have a plethora of tools in your toolbox to stay active and boost your mood.

# Misstep 3 Lack of intervals

As I mentioned above, too many people use steady-state cardio as their sole method of exercise, often because they have been drawn in by the "fat-burning-zone" feature on cardio equipment.

Don't buy into the idea that long bouts of mindless, easy cardio is the trick to losing weight and getting into shape. It isn't!

Now, steady, low-state endurance cardio (or fat-burning-zone cardio) is a fantastic first foray into working out, but if you are trying to lose fat, know that it doesn't lead to the level of fat loss that the name implies.

Fat-burning programs are based on the fact that working out at a lower intensity will burn a higher percentage of calories from fat. Yes, maintaining a lower heart rate will cause you to burn a higher percentage of calories from fat, but — this is important — because you are working at a lower intensity you will burn fewer calories overall. Opt for a program that challenges you to work at a higher intensity. Try interval training. You will burn a higher percentage of calories from carbohydrates, but since you burn more calories overall, you will create more of a metabolic demand on your body. Also, since you burn more calories overall, you are more likely to create a daily calorie deficit ("calorie deficit" means that you are burning more calories than you consume).

Both a high metabolic demand and a calorie deficit are needed for weight loss.

Plus, the term fat-burning zone elicits images of your adipose tissue (fat) magically disappearing off your hips. Instead, being in the fat-burning zone just means that you are using intra-muscular fat (the fat stored in your muscles) as fuel. That is a less enticing and less noticeable end result!

Don't be nervous about interval training. Intervals are not just for athletes; you can do intervals without running stairs or sprinting until you puke. Intervals simply mean that you alternate between bouts of higher- and lower-intensity activity. The intensity of your interval is dependent on your individual fitness level. For some, the high interval will be walking quickly. For others, it might be jogging.

Think of interval training as highway versus city driving. When you come off the highway, city driving seems slow, even though before you got on the highway, city driving didn't feel slow. It was your norm. Working at a higher level on a cardio machine, like driving faster while on the highway, teaches your body to understand that your normal is slow, and thus helps to increase your fitness.

The main take-away is, do some interval training, preferably two or three times a week. Interval training improves cardiovascular fitness, insulin sensitivity, and HDL (good) cholesterol, and helps reduce both visceral and subcutaneous fat. Visceral fat is the fat stored around your organs and subcutaneous fat is stored under your skin. These are the types of fat that lead to an expanding waistline and, particularly in the case of visceral fat, cause negative health consequences. (For "fun" interval workouts, check out chapter 10.)

# Misstep 4   Mindless eating and exercise habits

### Mindful eating 101

Too many people buy into what I call the "deserve mentality" — the "I went for a thirty-minute run today, so I deserve all the beer, cake, fried food, or (fill in the blank) that I want." I am not arguing that you should never have a beer — life is worth living. But if you are trying to lose weight, don't justify a day of mindless choices just because you worked out. Work out for the sake of feeling better and becoming fitter, not to eat copious amounts of food.

If you are exercising with the goal of losing weight, you have to be mindful of your nutrition and exercise choices. Many of us sabotage ourselves by misrepresenting reality. Don't tell yourself you had one helping of ice cream or a single beer if you actually had four helpings of ice cream in one big bowl or two beers in an oversized glass. The size of the bowl or the glass counts! Don't tell yourself you didn't eat dessert, or that you just had a "few" almonds, when in reality you ate cake off your partner's plate and grabbed massive handfuls of almonds off your colleague's desk throughout the day. Food counts, even when it is not on your plate.

Remember that exercise will help you lose weight only if none of the expended calories are replaced. In other words, exercise will help with weight loss only if you don't replace the calories you burned with extra food. So, have a treat if you want it, but understand that the treat will affect how quickly you reach your goal.

You might be surprised by how few calories you used during your workout and how many calories your "cheat" meal actually included. If you decide to indulge, be mindful of your portion and then enjoy the experience. Don't mindlessly eat, and don't use a workout as an excuse to binge. Portion sizes are always important, even on days you exercise.

Also, don't fall into the trap of believing that lifting weights and doing intervals a few times a week means you can be a sloth the rest of the time. Be mindful of your movement patterns throughout your entire week, not just at the gym. Prolonged sitting negatively affects the cardiovascular, lymphatic, and digestive systems, not to mention your metabolism. It is associated with increased risk of cardiovascular disease, stroke, and diabetes, and affects how your body metabolizes glucose. Move wherever and whenever possible.

### Limit costume-jewellery workouts

A client of mine coined the term "costume-jewellery workouts" to describe workouts where you just go through the motions — you might look like you are doing the real thing, but you aren't concentrating on what you are doing.

Basically, pay attention to your form; THINK about what you are doing! When you concentrate and become mindful of your movements, the quality of your workout will improve. Lack of awareness means that you simply strengthen muscles and reinforce neural pathways that are already strong.

Don't get me wrong; you don't need to be 100 percent present during every workout — especially cardio workouts.

If you are new to exercise, anything that will motivate you to exercise, including zoning out and exercising in front of the TV, is okay. Even exercise enthusiasts like me sometimes need a costume-jewellery workout. If I am in a crummy mood, I will often do a relaxed costume-jewellery run, where I am just going through the motions. The run gets my blood flowing, makes me feel productive, and ensures that I sleep well.

Just have enough awareness to know when you are doing the costume-jewellery version versus the real thing. To do a workout that will allow you to meet your goals, you have to know which type of workout you are doing.

When I do a relaxed run, I know that I am running to improve my mood, to get a break from my day, or as an active recovery workout. A costume-jewellery run is not in itself bad — it serves a purpose — as long as I don't kid myself. Costume-jewellery runs will not help me get a personal best, improve my fitness, or help me recruit underused muscles. If I am doing a specific speed workout, or strength exercises such as squats, I am very conscious of being mindful of my motions. I don't want to injure myself.

So, if you are recovering from an injury or attempting to retrain movement patterns (for example, changing your running gait or your squat form), it is important to make sure you are mindful. If you don't concentrate on what you are doing, you will simply reproduce your current muscle-recruitment patterns. If you are an experienced exerciser, running a few mindless five-kilometre runs will not help you lose weight, but if you are new to exercise, mindless cardio might be enough to help kick-start your workout routine.

Know what type of workout you are engaging in so that you can understand why you are — or are not — reaching your fitness goals.

# CHAPTER TAKE-AWAY

Stop relying on mindless cardio to get into shape. Do intervals, prioritize strength training, and make sure you recover appropriately. Become mindful of your exercise and nutritional habits so that you can accurately assess your habits and goals to determine why you are or are not achieving your goals. Be honest with yourself — assessing your health habits is pointless if you are consciously or unconsciously lying to yourself. Don't distort reality — misrepresenting reality leads to feelings of frustration and helplessness. Lying to yourself hurts only you. Own your choices!

# CHAPTER 10

# VARIETY IS THE SPICE OF LIFE

Don't become married to one activity — mix things up.
The world is your fitness oyster; never let yourself get bored.

So often people tell me that they stopped training out of boredom. Of course people quit training if they find it boring — disliking something is a huge disincentive! One of the reasons I love both my job and my own personal workouts is that training has limitless possibilities; there are always new ways to mix things up, new ways to "torture" and challenge my clients, new milestones to hit, new exercises to try, and new ways to make training fun. If you are thinking "Working out will never be fun. Kathleen is crazy," don't worry, I am used to that response. I am not offended. Let's compromise: If you don't believe working out will ever be "fun," at least mix things up so that your workouts are not mind-numbingly boring. No "auto-pilot" workouts allowed.

My mission in this chapter is to share some of those possibilities with you — to describe a variety of different workouts in the hope that you will discover one or two that you like (or at least don't hate), so that you are inspired to work out for the rest of your life.

Breathe new life into your workouts with one of the ideas below. As an added bonus, mixing up your workouts will help you avoid what is often referred to as a "fitness plateau" — the state where your body stops responding to the stimulus (workouts) that you have been giving it.

Trying a new workout serves multiple purposes; I get to work out, to explore when travelling, and to bond with whomever I am training with. For example, attending a class with my sister, Trissanna, is a nice excuse for us to get some sister time. She last visited me in the summer of 2015. During her visit we tried both a ballet-barre class and a Pilates class.

My best friend, Emily, and I try to go on one vacation together a year. Last time we went to Miami, where we did Pilates. With both Emily and Trissanna, the workouts were a bonding experience, an adventure, and a workout.

The moral is this: if you need some extra motivation, find a partner in crime. See chapter 7 for more information.

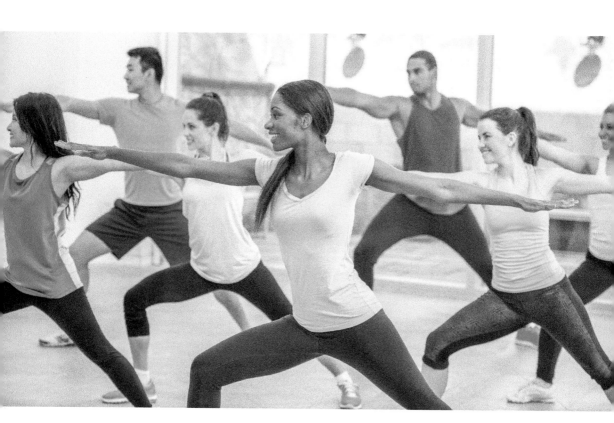

# Intervals

- - - - - - - - - - - - - - - - - - - - - - - - - - - - - - - - - - - - - - - - - - - - - - - - - - - - - - -

I love intervals. They are convenient — you can do them anywhere and on any piece of equipment or without equipment — AND they are effective. With intervals, you alternate between bouts of high- and low-intensity training. This places a high metabolic demand on the body, burns lots of calories in a short amount of time, produces a high EPOC (excess post-exercise oxygen consumption or, informally, "after-burn"), increases mitochondrial growth (mitochondria help to burn fat), and helps to improve one's fitness level. I find that keeping track of the time and shifting speeds makes my workout go by faster.

## Examples of Fun Intervals

Note: for all of the below workouts make sure you warm-up. A warm-up lasts between five and ten minutes and is basically a way to prepare your body for the more intense exercise to come. It is usually a scaled-down version of whatever you are going to do in the workout. For example,

Consider signing up for a running race and then incorporating intervals into your training. Having an established (and prepaid) goal can help you stay motivated, and the training can actually be fun. Plus, there is nothing like crossing a finish line; I always feel exhilarated and empowered when I do it.

First, pick the distance you want to complete. Then pick the date and location of the race so that you can train appropriately. The distance should match your level of fitness given how much time you have to prepare. Each week, aim to fit in a long run, a short recovery run, and one interval run. Determine the length of each run by the length of your race. So, for example, let's say you want to complete a ten-kilometre race. Once a week, do a long run that progressively increases in distance. Your long run should start at about six kilometres and you should work up to ten kilometres. Your second weekly run should be an easy five-kilometre run. Your third weekly run should be one of the interval workouts outlined in this chapter. It should be between four and eight kilometres.

my usual running speed is between an 8- and 9-minute mile, so I warm-up for five to ten minutes at a 10-minute mile. If you normally jog at an 11-minute mile then your warm-up might be a fast walk.

# Workout 1 Easy pick-ups

Warm up for five minutes. Do ten minutes at your regular speed (and regular level if you are on a machine that has levels), then cycle through the following pattern for ten minutes: alternate between thirty seconds at regular speed, twenty seconds slightly faster, and ten seconds fast. Finish with five to fifteen minutes at your regular speed and level. Cool down for five minutes.

# Workout 2 Pyramid intervals

With pyramid intervals the duration and/or intensity of the interval ramps either up or down throughout the workout.

## Version A
Warm up for five minutes. Then do one minute hard, one minute easy, two minutes hard, two minutes moderate, three minutes hard, three minutes moderate, four minutes hard, four minutes moderate, five minutes hard, one minute easy, and five minutes hard. Cool down for five to ten minutes.

## Version B
Warm up for five to ten minutes. Then cycle through the following sequence: thirty seconds hard, thirty seconds recovery, sixty seconds hard, sixty seconds recovery, ninety seconds hard, ninety seconds recovery. Repeat three to six times. Cool down for five to ten minutes.

# Workout 3 Mini pick-ups

Warm up for five minutes. Do five minutes at regular speed. Alternate fifteen seconds hard with forty-five seconds moderate for ten minutes. Recover for two minutes at regular speed. Then repeat the intervals by alternating fifteen seconds hard with forty-five seconds at regular speed. Cool down for five to eight minutes.

# Workout 4 Brick workout

A "brick" workout is where you do two different activities back to back with no rest. As a triathlete, I do brick workouts that combine swimming and biking or biking and running. You can use any two pieces of equipment. For example, use the rower and then the treadmill.

### Brick, part I

Do twenty minutes on any piece of equipment. Warm up for ten minutes. Do ten minutes at the hardest intensity you can hold.

### Brick, part 2

Immediately start your second activity — do five minutes of moderate work. Then do ten minutes at the hardest intensity you can hold. Finish with a five-minute cool-down.

If you do running intervals, remember that running is hard on the body. Every time you land, your support leg has to absorb the weight of your body, plus additional impact forces. Your entire kinetic chain has to be strong enough to support continuous single-leg impact forces far greater than just the weight of your body. If your kinetic chain is not strong enough or you don't give yourself enough recovery time between runs, injuries can occur.

Don't want to try intervals? No problem, try a non-interval brick workout. Do ten minutes on three different machines back to back. Regardless of what you try, remember: Never go from zero to one hundred. Progress gradually; let your muscles and connective tissue adapt.

"Kinetic chain" refers to an understanding of the body as more than individual muscles working independently, yet strung together. Instead, the body is understood as a chain of segments and joints; one motion creates a chain of events that affects the movement of neighbouring joints and muscles. This understanding of the body — as "chains" of muscles and joints — allows for a more functional interpretation of how the body moves. Within this functional conceptualization of movement, muscles don't work independently, they work as units. Think of that popular kids' song "the ankle bone is connected to the shin bone. The shin bone is connected to the knee bone" ... and so forth.

I hurt my hip in 2013 training for a half-marathon because I didn't appropriately ramp up my strength training or increase my recovery to mitigate the stress of the speed work I was doing. The capacity of my muscles was not sufficient to withstand the new stress of running at faster speeds.

Learn from my mistakes. If you decide to do running intervals, strength train and recover appropriately. Your strength always needs to be equal to or greater than what is demanded from the run.

# Mix Up Your Conditioning/Core/ Strength/Stretching Routines

. . . . . . . . . . . . . . . . . . . . . . . . . . . . . . . . . . . . . . . . . . . . . . . .

You don't have to do three sets of fifteen reps of the same four exercises or use machines for the rest of your life. Letting yourself get bored just sets you up for training failure. In this section, I have outlined a few alternative strength-training methods — time-based training and AMRAPs ("as many reps as possible") — and reviewed different types of fun group-exercise classes. Have a read and see if any of the workouts seem like something you would enjoy.

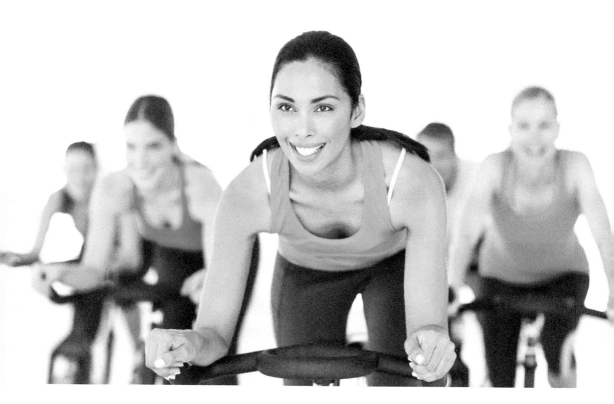

# Time-based training

Instead of structuring your workouts around attempting to complete a certain number of reps, do as many reps as you can in a certain amount of time. Try what I call "minutes" training.

## Minutes

Instead of doing an exercise for a pre-scribed number of reps, do as many reps as you can in one minute. Try three to ten exercises back to back for a minute each without any break. So, for example, after warming up, do one minute of squats, one minute of squat jumps, one minute of bridges, one minute of mountain climbers, and one minute of burpees all back to back without resting. Then take a one-minute rest and repeat two more times. Don't forget to cool down.

If you want more fun workout programs, take a look at my Pinterest page at www.pinterest.com/KTrotterFitness. I was inspired to create the page by a friend who said that she didn't want to make up her own plan, but that she also didn't trust a lot of the info online. She wanted the workout to be designed by me, so that she would know it was reliable. Now, whenever she wants — or if you want — a new "Kathleen-style" workout, there are always ones to pin. Enjoy!

Not sure what "mountain climbers" and burpees are? Think "plank with alternating knees in" and "a jumping plank." To do mountain climbers, start in a plank position, balancing on your hands and toes. Alternate "running" one knee into your chest at a time. For burpees, start standing, then bend over and place your hands on the floor, and jump your feet back into a plank. Hold for a moment. Then jump your feet back into your hands and stand or jump up.

## AMRAP training

AMRAP ("as many reps as possible") training is similar to minutes, but with AMRAP you aim to fit in as many cycles of a circuit as possible within a set time frame. The faster you get through the reps of each exercise, the more times you will complete the entire circuit in the given time frame. For example, try a six-minute AMRAP where you repeat twenty jumping jack and presses (a variation on a regular jumping jack where you press your arms over your head, with or without weights, as you do a jumping jack motion with your lower body), twenty lunges, and ten burpees as many times as you can in six minutes. Rest sixty to ninety seconds and then do another six-minute AMRAP of complementary exercises. For example, try ten push-ups, ten step-ups, and ten bent-over rows. Aim for three to five six-minute AMRAP sets separated by sixty to ninety seconds of rest per workout.

Or try a "work/rest" AMRAP. Decide on a time frame — let's say two minutes — then pick three to four exercises that you can complete in roughly one and a half minutes. The workout looks like this: You have two minutes to complete the four exercises. If you complete them in a minute and a half, you get thirty seconds' rest. If you complete them in a minute and forty-five seconds, you get fifteen seconds' rest. Do five to six sets all the way through. By the end,

it should be a challenge to fit the exercises into the two-minute time frame.

AMRAP workouts are effective and efficient workouts because they burn lots of calories in a short period of time, plus they provide a high EPOC, which is the number of calories you burn after the workout is over. I encourage my clients to try them because they can be done using a wide range of equipment If you are at home, do body-weight exercises like squats and burpees. If you are at the gym, use the barbell, cable machines, or Bosu. A Bosu looks almost like a half ball, with a platform on one side and an inflatable dome on the other. It adds an element of instability to many exercises, such as burpees or V-sits, to challenge your balance and increase the difficulty.

No injuries allowed — only include exercises in your AMRAP that you can do with perfect form.

## Pilates

Pilates strengthens the core and improves posture, and since mat Pilates doesn't require equipment, you can do it anywhere. Get yourself a Pilates DVD and bring it along when you travel.

If possible, find a class with an appropriate teacher-to-student ratio so that the teacher can watch your form, and a knowledgeable instructor who prioritizes

## Bridge

At home try the bridge, a staple of most Pilates classes.

Lie on your back, feet shoulder-width apart. Use your bum to lift your hips, then lower them back to the floor. At the end of twenty reps, hold your hips up and pulse them twenty times. Don't push with your lower back, use your bum. To give yourself a challenge, place a small, squishy ball (you can buy one at the dollar store) under your feet as you lift your hips up and down twenty times. Try not to wobble.

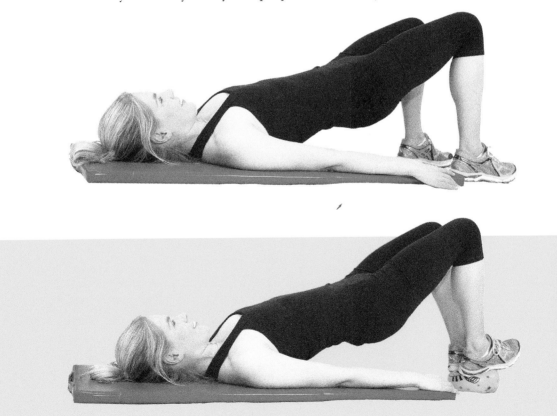

exercises that strengthen all the small stabilizer muscles of the foot, knee, core, upper back, and neck, and limits forward flexion exercises. Many instructors prioritize exercises — like the hundreds and the roll-up — that require forward flexion or crunching forward. Performing exercises where you crunch forward, without equal or greater amounts of exercises that promote spinal extension, like "swimming," can contribute to a rounded-forward posture. I also find that too often instructors speed through the explanation and execution of the exercises; they don't take the time to properly explain form, and their tempo is more appropriate to that of a dance or aerobics class than a Pilates class. Most Pilates exercises — at least initially — should be done slowly, with purpose and conscious thought.

Pilates movements, when done correctly, are subtle. If you think you are doing something wrong, ask. There is no point in reinforcing bad form.

## Yoga

Different types of yoga offer slightly different benefits. A restorative or Hatha class will offer greater relaxation benefits, whereas an Ashtanga class is more vigorous and involves more weight-bearing exercises, making it a better substitute for weight training.

That said, whether yoga is the most ideal workout for you depends on your flexibility.

A balance of flexibility and strength is needed for optimum muscular and joint function.

When it comes to stretching, more is NOT always better. Too much mobility can be detrimental. Think ankle sprains and dislocated shoulders. Excessive flexibility, without the corresponding strength, can lead to unstable joints.

Strength without flexibility, on the other hand, can lead to muscles that become strained from something as simple as bending down to tie your shoes.

If you are naturally flexible, prioritize traditional strength exercises. Aim for a three-to-one ratio of strength-to-flexibility activities. If you do yoga, don't "hang out in your joints" — meaning don't lock your joints, especially your knees and elbows, to give you support. Focus on using your muscles to support your joints; when you consciously use your muscles you are more likely to get the strength-building benefits of yoga.

If you are strong and relatively inflexible, prioritize yoga, but don't yank or bounce in the pose. Aim for a three-to-one ratio of flexibility-to-strength workouts.

Remember, the best type of exercise program will differ from person to person. It is a unique combination of what is affordable, realistic, and convenient; what the individual likes to do; and what the individual should do to fix their body's "weak links."

If you can afford it, invest in a few one-on-one or semi-private sessions. Yoga classes in general can be dangerous for beginners. It can be hard for the instructor to get to everyone, owing to the sheer volume of participants.

Many people love hot yoga, but hot yoga is not appropriate for beginners. Participants should be familiar with traditional yoga (or at least other forms of flexibility-based exercise), so that they have the mind-body awareness to know what an appropriate range of motion for their body is.

When stretching, as you approach the limits of your flexibility, your body provides a pain response. This pain response is a good thing — it tells you how far you can safely stretch without injuring yourself. Heat delays the pain response, allowing you to stretch farther.

That may sound like a good thing; in fact, people often go to hot yoga for that very reason. The problem is, heat doesn't actually make you more flexible, it just delays the pain response, thus making it more likely that you will overstretch and hurt yourself.

If you decide you want to go to hot yoga, participate in some regular yoga classes first to figure out your personal limits. Then, when you go to hot yoga, work within those limits. Don't be seduced by your ego or a teacher encouraging you to "go deeper." Stop stretching before you feel pain, not when you feel pain.

## Spin

I am a fan of spin — a high-intensity fitness class on a stationary bike — because it usually includes intervals, which I think are important. The act of alternating between periods of high- and low-intensity activity burns lots of calories, results in a relatively high EPOC (post-exercise calorie burn), and burns fat. Plus, intervals can vastly improve a person's fitness level; what you originally considered a challenge, or your "intense" interval, gradually becomes your new baseline, or "recovery" interval. Spin is also non–weight bearing, which is a positive if you are looking for low-impact activities (for example, if you have osteoarthritis).

That said, spin classes can be expensive, plus you have to spend time getting to and from the studio. So a forty-five-minute class can turn into a two-hour time commitment. I have a bike at home, so not only is a forty-five-minute workout free, it also actually only takes forty-five minutes. Most people don't have spin bikes in their homes, which means spin becomes unrealistic financially, and too big of a time commitment. Also, because spin is non–weight bearing, it doesn't strengthen bones and help to prevent osteoporosis. If you spin, also walk and strength train regularly to increase your bone density.

Spinning also involves sitting, and usually a fair amount of bending forward, which can create stiffness in the hips and back and promote bad posture. To counteract the strain of sitting on the bike (especially because sitting is something most of us do way too much already), prioritize flexibility exercises that mobilize the hips and chest, and strength exercises that strengthen the upper back and core.

Last, make sure your bike is properly set up and that you always have resistance on your fly wheel, especially when spinning quickly. Stay in control and prioritize proper form — quality over quantity!

## Ballet barre

Barre classes allow participants to train like dancers while using light weights, resistance bands, the barre, and a squishy ball. Barre promotes flexibility and joint mobility, which many of us need since we all tend to sit too much. When we do move, it is often in set forward-movement patterns (walking, biking, elliptical, and running). Lack of movement or repetitive patterns (like running) can cause stiffness and often result in certain muscles becoming stronger than others.

So, if you sit a lot or your current exercise routine includes repetitive activities like running (like me, hence why I benefit from the class), this class might complement your lifestyle.

That said, classes are expensive and can be inconvenient to get to. Ballet barre is a fairly new phenomenon; currently classes are mostly offered at small boutique studios. As they get more popular, I am sure that mainstream gyms will start offering them, which will make them more cost-effective.

Another possible negative is that ballet-barre classes don't have a large amount of potential for long-term progressive overload. This is a training theory that states that to continue to progress, you have to constantly challenge the body. Since the class relies on small weighted balls, the resistance band, and your body weight, a ceiling of possible overload exists, but unless you wear a weighted vest or bring dumbbells to the class, the overload that the balls, band, and your body weight can provide is limited.

The limited overload is fine if you are a beginner or if you plan to mix in other activities, but don't make ballet barre your sole method of training for a sustained period of time. If you already do mobility-based classes like yoga, if you participate in sports that require you to move in multiple directions (think soccer), or if your goal is pure muscular strength, traditional strength workouts might be a better fit.

Last, always remember that although barre is marketed on the idea that doing the routine will get you a dancer's body, the studio is trying to sell a product. A dancer's body is a product of their genetics, their lifestyle, the sheer volume of hours they

## Barre Series

Try this barre series at home. Most of you probably don't have a barre in your living room — I know I don't — so just use a countertop or the back of a chair.

- Place your hands lightly on your makeshift barre. Hinge at your waist. Don't round your back. Use your core to support your weight. Make sure you are not hollowing out your midsection or simply "sucking in" your stomach to do this. Instead, start by engaging your pelvic floor. Then, gently pull your belly button to your spine while you simultaneously try to activate your lower abdominals. To activate your lower abdominals, imagine you are pulling your lower abdominals wide to your hip bones. Another helpful image is to imagine you are "putting on a slightly tight pair of pants, and thus you have to pull your low abdominals gently away from the pants." Engage the bum muscles of your left leg to support your body.
- Turn your right thigh bone out and then bring your right leg backward fifteen times. Use your bum, not your lower back.
- After fifteen reps, hold your leg up behind you and pulse it ten times. Finish by making ten little circles with your leg in each direction. Keep your core stable as you move your leg. Imagine you are holding a plank position. Switch sides and repeat with your left leg.

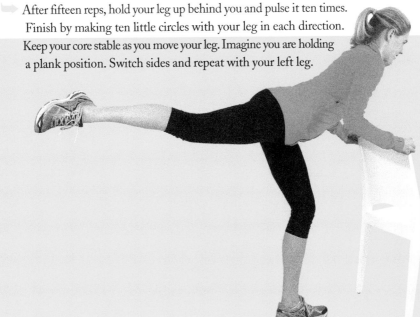

train, and impeccable nutrition. Absolutely try a ballet-barre class — it is a great work-out — but have realistic expectations.

## CrossFit

I appreciate the importance that CrossFit places on functional multi-joint exercises like squats, deadlifts, bench presses, and pull-ups. That said, CrossFit is not for every "body."

Is it for you? That depends on your personality, fitness level, past and present injuries, budget, goals, and desired gym atmosphere.

CrossFit gyms ("boxes") vary in size and amenities, but they are usually in warehouse-like facilities that contain virtually no traditional machines. Instead, they are filled with equipment such as barbells, dumbbells, kettlebells, and medicine balls. If you think you would like this "back to basics" environment, then CrossFit may be for you.

CrossFit is not cheap. The facilities are not fancy. You pay for the intensity of the workouts and the non-traditional aspect of the gym. If you want a fancier gym, CrossFit is not for you.

The workouts are advanced. Again, this can be a positive or a negative. The CrossFit websites I read state that people of all fitness levels are welcome, but the competitive atmosphere that these gyms foster, although motivating, doesn't make it easy to scale back a workout.

All members are encouraged to work toward achieving PBs (personal bests). In theory, this type of goal setting is fantastic, but since participants write their results on a public board, some people may have a hard time scaling back their workouts to an appropriate level.

Also, since the exercises start at an advanced level, the scaled-back version might still be too advanced for some people. This can be a recipe for injury, which is compounded by the fact that many new lifters don't yet know their limits.

If you decide to try a class, be careful. Listen to your body. Stop if something feels wrong. If your CrossFit gym offers an introductory course (most do, although not all of them make it mandatory), take it. Every CrossFit gym and coach is slightly different. Shop around. Try different places and teachers until you find a combo that is a good fit.

Whatever class you try — whether it is spin, barre, CrossFit, or something else — remember these words: You have to earn the right to progress. Meaning, before you try a new exercise, or increase the amount of weight you are lifting, make sure you have mastered the basic version and have, therefore, earned the right to progress. Progress gradually. You have to put in the work to be able to do harder exercises, use heavier weights, or run for longer. Asking yourself if you have earned your progression regularly will help you avoid injury.

### Deadlifts

A popular CrossFit exercise is deadlifts. I love deadlifts because they strengthen the core, glutes, and lower back. Most of us have a chronically weak core and bum from sitting too much. But deadlifts are easy to do incorrectly. Make sure you perfect your form before you challenge yourself with extra weight.

➤ Start by standing with feet slightly wider than shoulder-width apart. Hold two dumbbells, arms at your side, palms facing you, shoulders back, core engaged, and chest out.

➤ Start by hinging at your hips. Don't round your back. Once the weights pass your knees, bend your knees so that the dumbbells continue to move toward the floor. At the bottom, power with your hips and core so that you explode back to standing. Start by doing a moderate rep scheme with a light weight. Once you have perfected your form, play around with doing multiple sets of fewer reps at a heavier weight. For example, try four sets of six to eight reps.

➤ Use your bum, hamstrings, and lower back and make sure to keep your back straight. A rounded back is a dead giveaway that someone has lost their form.

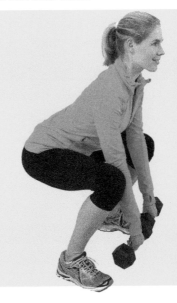

# CHAPTER TAKE-AWAY

Don't let yourself fall into a fitness rut. Experiment: if you always run, try spinning. If you always take yoga classes, try a pump class or a Pilates class.

If you try a workout and you don't like it, no problem; maybe you can still learn something from the experience. For example, if you don't end up loving CrossFit but you like a few of the strength exercises, incorporate them into your routine.

If you like the format of a class, but don't love the teacher, shop around until you find someone that you like. I have tried over ten versions of ballet barre. I loved a few of them, tolerated a few, and outright disliked another.

Basically, keep trying different workout adventures until you find something you like.

To quote the late-eighties fitness show *BodyBreak* — remember to "keep fit and have fun."

# CHAPTER 11

# THE "CHOOSE YOUR OWN ADVENTURE" EXERCISE PROGRAM

Don't try to fit a square peg into a round hole.

Stop trying to adapt your lifestyle to fit generic, pre-set fitness routines. Other people's regimens are exactly that — theirs! Sure, you can twist yourself into knots and adapt to someone else's program for a few weeks, but chances are you won't be able to or won't want to maintain the program over the long haul.

Instead of looking for a miracle plan to follow, develop your own recipe for success. Put together a program that is realistic, sustainable, and built around your unique reality, rhythms, lifestyle, and personal goals.

# How to Build Your Unique Recipe

. . . . . . . . . . . . . . . . . . . . . . . . . . . . . . . . . . . . . . . . . . . . . . . . .

First, answer the questions below to determine your exercise personality. Then use the specific guidelines to create your program.

What type of exercise personality do you have?

Are you a gym bunny, competitive athletic gym bunny, time-crunched multitasker, or homebody?

Do you find designated workout areas — like the gym — motivating? Do you need lots of different equipment to stay into your workout? Do you get bored and lose motivation if you aren't constantly changing up your workout? Do you enjoy being with others when you train? Do you thrive off friendly competition?

If so, then you are what I would call a gym bunny.

If you answered yes to all the questions, and an emphatic YES to the final two questions, then you are what I would call a competitive athletic gym bunny, which means you enjoy the structured nature of the gym as well as friendly competition and athletic activities.

Do you always feel too busy to work out? Do you feel rushed from one appointment to another and pulled in a million different directions by your family, friends, and job? Do you know that exercise is good for you but can't contemplate getting yourself to the gym or a structured exercise class?

If so, you are a time-crunched multitasker. Meaning that, at least for now, life has to be your gym. Build movement into your life and turn activities you already do into workouts.

Do you hate the vibe of most gyms and dislike working out in front of people, but still want a somewhat structured routine? Do you lack the patience to waste time getting to and from the gym, but still want a fairly intense workout?

If you answered yes, you are a homebody. You want a vigorous workout without having to get to the gym. Lucky for you, you can get an intense, full-body workout in the comfort of your home gym.

# The Gym Bunny Program

Do cardio three to five days per week. Use any cardio machine, run or bike outside, or try a group-exercise class such as spin, aerobics, or dance.

Make sure that two to three days per week your cardio workouts are intervals.

## Sample cardio workout

Pick a cardio machine — any machine will do. Warm up for ten minutes. Cycle through: thirty seconds hard, thirty seconds recovery, sixty seconds hard, sixty seconds recovery, ninety seconds hard, ninety seconds recovery. Repeat three to six times. Cool down for five minutes. (See chapter 10 for other interval workouts.)

Strength train two or three times per week. Try a group weight-training class and/or try the workout below. Strength train on non-consecutive days, and remember to experiment — one week, try ballet barre. The next week, try Pilates. (See chapter 10 for additional group-exercise options.)

## Sample strength workout

Complete two sets of each circuit. To complete one circuit, do all exercises within that circuit back to back without resting. At the end of the circuit, rest for thirty seconds and repeat. Pick a weight that allows you to do all of the repetitions with good form but that you find challenging during the last few repetitions.

Going forward, complete three sets of each circuit. Challenge yourself by lifting heavier weights and/or try the "kick it up a notch" modification. All exercises and modifications can be found in the "Exercise Descriptions" section of this chapter.

## CIRCUIT 1

⇒ Machine rows: twelve to fifteen reps

⇒ Squats: twelve to fifteen reps

⇒ Standing stability-ball sweeps: ten reps each side

## CIRCUIT 2

⇒ Lat pull-down machine: twelve to fifteen reps

⇒ *Straight-arm lat pull-down: twelve to fifteen reps

⇒ Lunges: twelve to fifteen reps each leg

*Use the bar on the lat pull-down machine or the cable machine.

## CIRCUIT 3

⇒ Windshield wipers with band or towel: twelve to fifteen reps

⇒ Bird dog: six reps each side

⇒ Front plank: hold for twenty seconds or longer

⇒ Side plank: hold for twenty seconds or longer

## STRETCHES

⇒ Standing calf stretch: hold for at least thirty seconds each leg

⇒ Figure-four stretch: hold for at least thirty seconds each leg

⇒ Standing lunge hip-flexor stretch: hold for at least thirty seconds each leg

⇒ Hamstring stretch: hold for at least thirty seconds each leg

⇒ Door-Frame chest stretch: hold for at least thirty seconds each arm

# CIRCUIT I

**Machine Rows:**

➡ Face the cable machine. Sit up straight, core engaged. Use your upper back (not your biceps) to pull the bar toward your chest. Hold for a moment — imagine that you are cracking a walnut with your shoulder blades — and then slowly release.

**Kick it up a notch with standing single-arm cable rows:**

➡ Stand facing the cable machine in a staggered stance, right leg forward. The cable should be roughly at chest height. Grab the D-handle with your right hand, arm straight out in front of you. Bend your left arm and tuck your elbow into your side. This is your starting position. Row your right arm back as you press your left arm forward, like you are using a bow and arrow. Return your arms to their starting position. Initiate the row with your upper back. Use your torso muscles to twist.

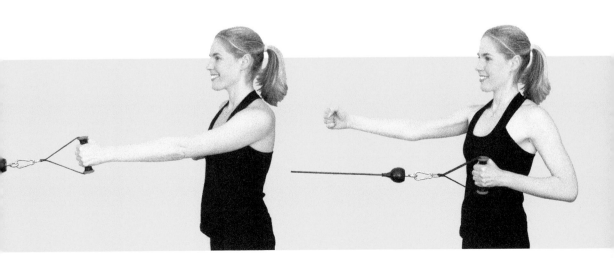

### Squats

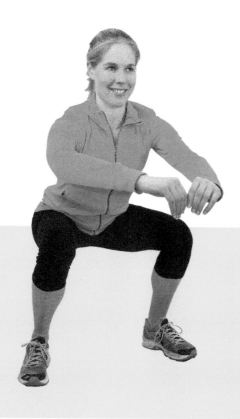 Start with your feet shoulder-width apart and parallel. Bend at your ankles, knees, and hips to sit your bum backward, like you are sitting down into a chair. At the bottom, engage your bum and core to push yourself up to standing.

**Kick it up a notch:**

Hold free weights at your shoulders.

Tip: Don't just plunk yourself down. Control your body on the way down — imagine that someone is pushing you down and you are resisting the push.

## Standing Stability-Ball Sweeps

➡ Stand on your right leg holding a stability ball by the outside of your right hip. Sweep the ball up over your left shoulder so that the ball almost touches your left ear. Your right bum muscles should be working, and both hip bones should remain facing forward as the ball moves.

Kick it up a notch:

➡ Close your eyes or stand on a Bosu.

Tip: Look ahead, not down.

# CIRCUIT 2

### Lat Pull-Down

➥ Grab the bar slightly wider than shoulder-width apart and sit facing the lat pull-down machine. Hinge backward about five degrees, but don't let your lower back arch. Engage your core. Hinge from your hips, not your lower back. Pull the bar down by initiating the movement from your upper back and — this is key — don't round forward as you pull the bar down. If your shoulders round forward, you are engaging more of your chest and shoulders and less of your back. Hold the bar at your chest for one count, then slowly straighten your arms. Don't let the weight pull your arms — control the motion with your muscles.

**Kick it up a notch:**

➥ Add a two-second hold at the bottom of the motion.

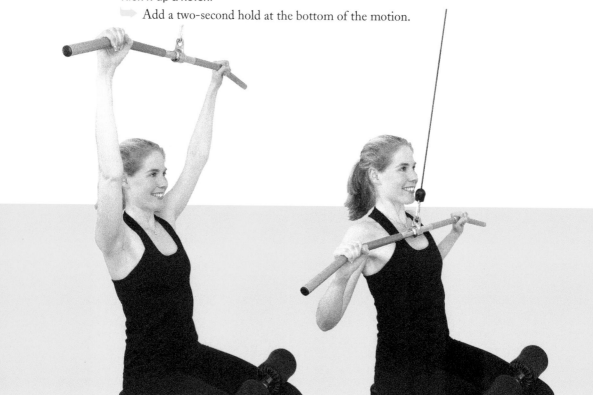

### Straight-Arm Lat Pull-Downs

Stand facing the pull-down machine. Hold the bar shoulder-width apart, palms down, arms straight. Keep them straight throughout the entire motion. First, draw the upper portion of your humerus (the long bone in the upper arm between the elbow joint and shoulder) back in your shoulder sockets and engage your core. Then, keeping the top of your humerus back, pull the bar down to your thighs. Don't round forward as you pull the bar down. Slowly release.

### Kick it up a notch

Add a two-second hold at the bottom of the motion.

Tip: As you pull the bar down, imagine that a piece of string is pulling your chest up toward the ceiling.

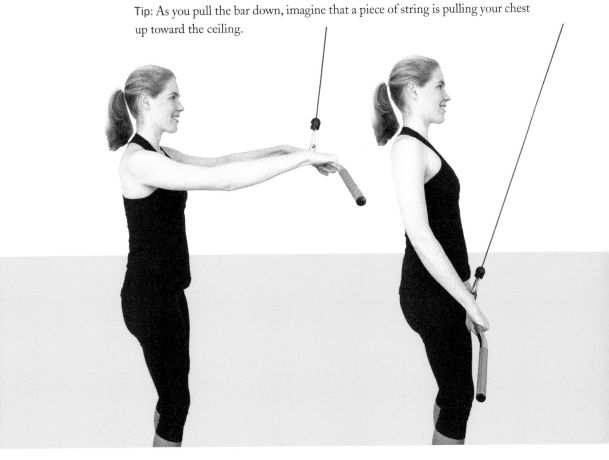

## Lunges

Start standing, both feet facing forward. Step your right leg back. Bend both knees so that your body lowers toward the floor. Don't let your front knee go forward over your front toes — keep your front heel on the ground. Hold at the bottom for one count. Then engage the left bum muscle to push yourself up to standing. Switch legs.

**Kick it up a notch:**

Hold weights and/or add a hold at the bottom of the motion for two to four seconds.

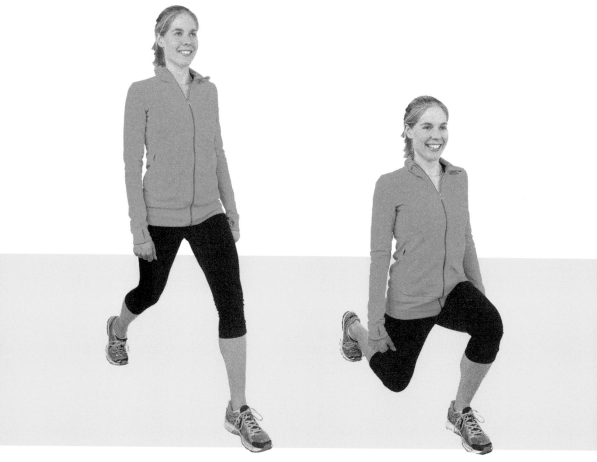

## CIRCUIT 3

### Windshield Wipers

You will need a towel for this. Stand with your elbows at your sides, arms bent at a ninety-degree angle. Hold the towel so that it is horizontal to the floor, your palms up. Draw the upper portion of your humerus (arm bone) backward into your shoulder sockets. Then feel the muscles around your right shoulder blade work to rotate your right hand out to the right. Resist the rotation with the muscles around your left shoulder blade. Without resting, use the muscles around your left shoulder blade to rotate the towel to the left. Resist the motion with your right arm. Both arms should always be working — it is a continuous motion. One arm pulls while the other arm resists — your arms should look somewhat like windshield wipers.

### Bird Dog

Start on your hands and knees, hands under your shoulders and knees under your hips. Distribute your weight evenly between all four of your limbs. Without shifting, straighten and raise your right arm and left leg so they are level with the floor. Keep your right leg straight and use your core. Return to the starting position and switch sides. To make sure you are using correct form, place a water bottle on your back. Don't let it fall off as you move.

Kick it up a notch:

When your arm is extended, write your name in the air with your hand. To make it even harder, add an arm rotation. Start by extending your right arm and left leg. Then keep your leg extended as your reach your right arm out to your side and twist toward the ceiling. The twist should come from your ribs, not just from your arm.

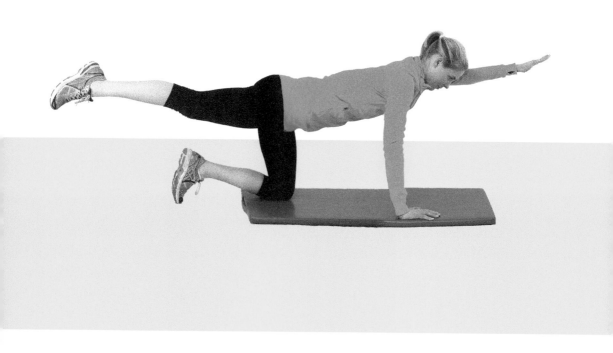

### Front Plank

➡ Place your forearms and either your knees or the tips of your toes on the ground. Then lift your body off the mat so that only your forearms and either your knees or toes are touching the floor. Make sure that your bum is not up in the air, your upper back is not hunched, and your lower back is not arched. Your body should look like a plank. Once you can easily do a minute from your knees, balance on your toes. When you transition from a modified (knee) plank to a plank from your toes, initially decrease the time you hold the position.

### Kick it up a notch:

➡ Hold your plank for longer and/or do plank scapula retractions. In the plank position, pull your shoulder blades together ten to fifteen times. Don't arch or round your back. Imagine that you are trying to crack a walnut with your shoulder blades.

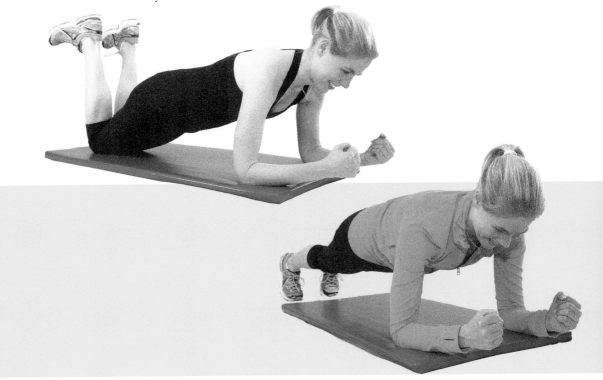

### Side Plank

Start by lying on your side with your forearm on the ground in front of you. Lift up and balance on one forearm and either your knees or the outside edge of your foot. Keep your core engaged and don't round through your upper back. Draw your top shoulder backward and make sure your rib cage is not jutting forward. If it is, pull your rib cage backward so that it is in line with your pelvis. Once you can easily hold this position for a minute on your knees, do the exercise from the outside edge of your foot. When you transition from a modified plank to a plank from your toes, slightly decrease the time you hold the position.

**Kick it up a notch:**

Hold your side plank for longer and/or add a side leg lift. Hold yourself in the side plank position as you lift your top leg up and then lower it. Use the bum muscles of the leg closest to the ceiling to lift the leg up and to lower, and the bum muscles of your bottom leg to hold your body up. Keep your pelvis stable. Initially, do this exercise from your knees. It is challenging.

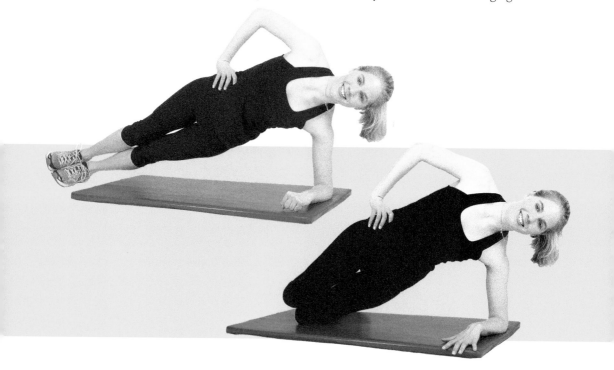

## STRETCHES

### Standing Calf Stretch

➡ Stand with your forearms against a wall, one leg back, one leg forward, both feet facing forward. Push your pelvis forward, keep your back heel down and back leg straight. Hold for a minimum of thirty seconds. Switch and repeat.

### Figure-Four Stretch

➡ Sit tall in a chair, shoulders back. Look ahead as you cross your right ankle over your left knee. Push gently on your right thigh. Feel the stretch in the outside of the right hip. Hold for thirty seconds and repeat on the opposite side.

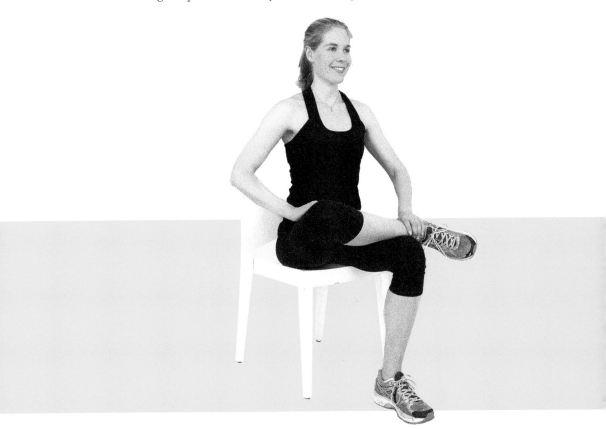

### Standing Lunge Hip-Flexor Stretch

Step your right leg behind you. Keep both feet facing forward and bend your knees slightly. Tuck your pelvis so that your right hip bone moves toward your ribs. Feel the stretch up the front of your right thigh. Hold for thirty seconds before switching legs.

### Hamstring Stretch

Lie on your back. Grab the upper thigh of your right leg, straighten the leg, and pull it up toward your chest. It is more important to keep the right leg straight than to bring it to the chest. Hold for a minimum of thirty seconds. Then switch legs and repeat.

### Door-Frame Chest Stretch

Place the forearm of one arm against the edge of a door frame at roughly chest height. Your arm should be bent at a ninety-degree angle. Turn your body gently away from the arm so that you feel a slight stretch in your chest and shoulders. Hold for thirty seconds. Switch and repeat with the opposite arm.

# The Competitive Athletic Gym Bunny Program

Follow the same program as the gym bunny, but replace one weekly cardio workout with a sport: join a basketball or soccer team or even a running group — anything that fosters some friendly competition and allows you to be social. Also, consider replacing one of your solo weight workouts with something more collaborative. Try a competitive class like CrossFit, join a conditioning program for athletes, or simply make a few friends who will lift weights with you.

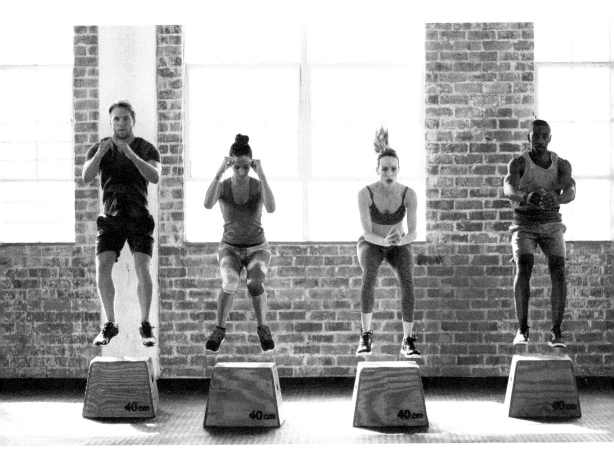

# The Time-Crunched Multi-Tasker Program

Think of your daily life as your gym — find ways to weave motion into everything you do. Every bit of motion adds up, and every situation can be reframed as an opportunity for movement.

## Fartlek Intervals

Three days per week, do at least twenty minutes of fartlek intervals while you walk. Fartlek intervals are challenging but unstructured, so you get a great interval workout without having to constantly look at your watch. Warm up for five minutes, then pick a random landmark — such as a stop sign — and speed walk, run, or sprint toward it. Walk or jog to recover. Repeat until it is time to go home. Make sure to budget for a five-minute cool-down.

## Piggyback Strategy

Try the piggyback strategy of turning things you already do into a workout.

- Don't do work as you sit waiting for your child to complete her after-school activity; bring your exercise clothes and use that hour to go for a walk or run. If you want to watch your child's practice or game, do squats and lunges on the sidelines. Bring a mat to do floor work or wrap a resistance band around a tree to do a set of rows, or stand on it to do bicep curls.
- Pace while on conference calls.
- Brainstorm with colleagues while walking instead of over a meal or drinks.
- Bike to and from work.
- Walk your children to school and then run home.
- Walk or jog with your dog. Even better, stop at the dog park mid-walk or jog and throw a ball; while your dog is fetching it, do jumping jacks and lunges.
- Make family fun time active. In the summer, go for bike rides or hikes. In the winter, try skiing or skating.
- Dance around your living room as you watch TV.
- Make active dates with your partner or spouse.

## Weave in strength, balance, and core exercises throughout your day

Aim to do at least five posture-friendly exercises daily. They can be done anywhere — in your kitchen, at work, or waiting for an elevator.

### POSTURE-FRIENDLY EXERCISES
#### Standing Side Leg Lifts

Stand on one leg on the edge of a step, yoga block, or book. Engage the bum muscles of the standing leg. Make sure the weight in your support foot is even. Don't lean as you kick the other leg out to the side. Hold the kick out to the side for one to two seconds. Do ten to fifteen reps. Then switch and repeat on the other leg.

### Drunk Walks

Start standing. Place your right heel in front of your left toes as if you were walking on a tightrope. Your feet should make a straight line. Take three steps along the rope. Don't look down. After three steps, pause and make sure that your shoulders are back, your core is engaged, and you are looking straight ahead. Then close your eyes. Maintain the position of your body. Don't fall over. Open your eyes and continue. Repeat for six to ten reps.

### Wall Push

Stand with your back against the wall, knees slightly bent, arms straight, and palms facing the wall. Your palms should be gently touching the wall, but don't get distracted by your hand placement. The motion is about moving your shoulder blades. Yes, your hands will push slightly into the wall, but only because your shoulder blades and your upper back are initiating the motion. Pull your shoulder blades back, tuck your chin like you are trying to give yourself a double chin, and simultaneously push into the wall with your hands. Don't arch your lower back as you push into the wall. Hold for five seconds. Release and repeat ten times.

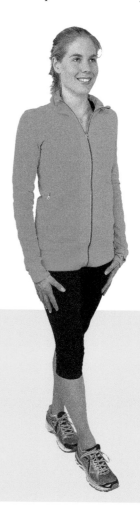

### Seated Twist

➡ Sit tall in your chair. Reach your left hand across your body so that it sits on the outside of your right knee. Use your left hand to pull GENTLY on your right knee so that you rotate to the right. Hold for fifteen seconds and then switch sides. Do one to three twists each side.

### Seated Core Work

➡ A strong core will help your posture. Start by bringing your bum close to the edge of your chair. Keep your back straight and lean backward roughly ten degrees. Hold for ten seconds to a minute. Aim to do as many reps as needed until the total time held is one minute. The bonus of getting stronger is that once you can hold the exercise for one minute, you only have to do it once.

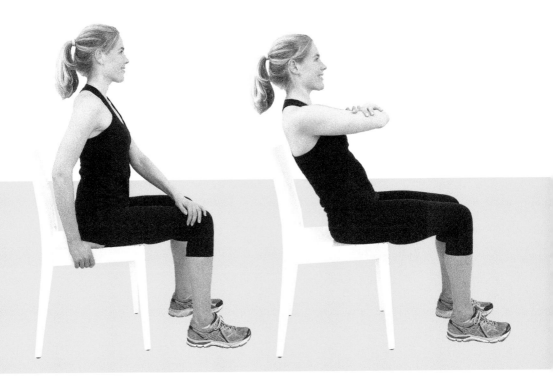

### Upper-Back Massage with a Tennis Ball

Stand with your upper back against the wall, with the ball between your back and the wall. Press your body into the ball, and move your body up and down so that the ball massages your entire back. When you feel a tender spot, hold and breathe into it for ten seconds. If you have a yoga tune-up ball, use it.

### Wall Ys to Ws

Stand with your bum and back against a wall, core engaged, legs shoulder-width apart, knees slightly bent, and feet roughly half a foot in front of the wall. You should be able to fit your fingers, but not your entire hand, between your lower spine and the wall. Form a W with your arms. Keep your arms as close to the wall as you can while you straighten them until they form a Y with your body. Make sure that your spine stays neutral. It shouldn't arch as you move your arms, even if that means the back of your hands move away from the wall. Return your arms to the W position and repeat five to ten times.

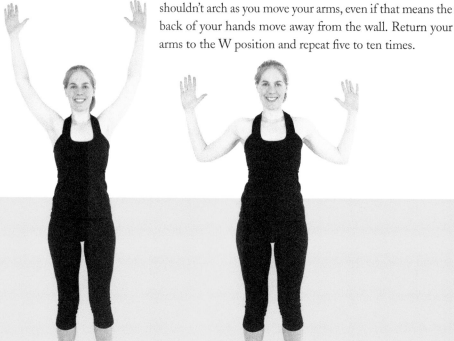

### Wrist Wall Walks

→ Face a wall and lift your arms up to chest height. Keep your arms straight as you place the back of your hands against the wall, fingers down. Maintain this hand position as you "walk" your hands up the wall four or five times. Return your hands to their starting position and change your hand placement — put your palms against the wall, fingers up. Again, walk your hands up the wall. Step away from the wall, gently rotate your wrists ten times clockwise, followed by ten times counter-clockwise. Don't force anything. All of the steps should feel good. Repeat for five to ten reps on each hand.

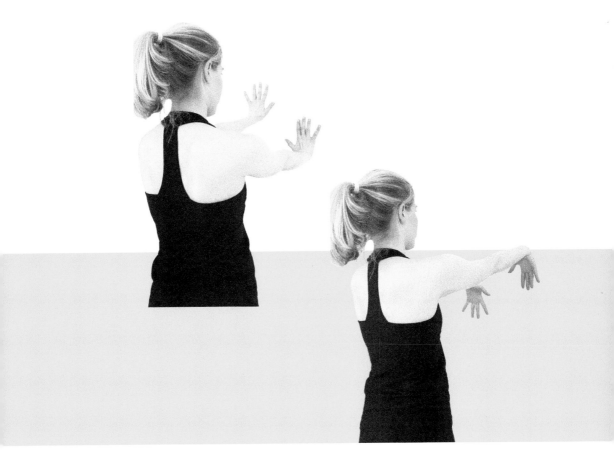

### Standing Upper-Back Door-Frame Stretch

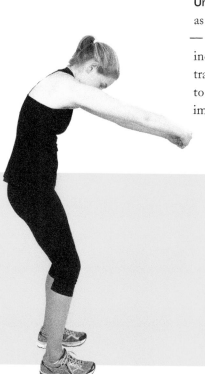

Grip a door frame with both hands. Sit your hips backward and round through your upper back. Resist the pull with your hands. Hold for fifteen to thirty seconds.

### Shoulder, Elbow, Arm Rotations

This exercise has three parts. Start with your arms by your side. To do part one, keep your hands by your side and simply roll your shoulders backward. To do part two, lift your arms up and lead with your elbows to roll your shoulders back. This will mean your elbows will point back behind you as you roll your shoulders. To complete part three, straighten your arms and make a big circle backward with your arms. Try to feel your shoulder blades move as you do all three actions. Repeat the cycle five times. See chapter 3 and the Gym Bunny Program in this chapter for additional stretches.

**One final note:** Think of this multi-tasker program as an interim program. As your schedule changes — even if that is not until you retire — aim to include structured workouts, especially weight training, more frequently. Lifting weights helps to decrease the likelihood of osteoporosis and improves your functional fitness.

# The Homebody Program

. . . . . . . . . . . . . . . . . . . . . . . . . . . . . . . . . . . . . . . . . . . . . . . . . . . . . .

Two to three times per week, do at least twenty minutes of cardio. Walk or jog outside, dance around your living room, skip rope, ride your bike, or use your stairs.

## Sample homebody workout I

Walk up and down the stairs for five minutes and then do five minutes of high knees, bum kicks, jumping jacks, and running or walking on the spot to warm up. To do high knees, start standing and alternate bringing one knee up toward the ceiling at a time. For a low-impact workout, simply lift the knees as high as you can, making sure one foot stays on the floor at all times. For a higher-impact workout, "run" your knees up toward your chest. This means there will be moments where you are switching feet in midair. For bum kicks, stand and alternate kicking your bum with your heel. Again, for a low impact workout, keep one foot on the floor at all times. For a higher-impact workout, "run" your heels toward your bum. To do a jumping jack, stand with your hands by your sides and your feet together. Jump your feet wide as you bring your arms up over your head. Jump your feet back together as you lower your arms. Repeat. For a low-impact version, simply alternate tapping one foot out to the side at a time.

Once you have warmed-up, walk up the stairs once, jog up the stairs once, and then run up the stairs once. (If running is too intense, jog instead.) Walk, jog, or run in place for one minute. Repeat that cycle for ten minutes. Each week, add on one minute of work until you can do twenty to thirty minutes of the cycle. Cool down for five minutes. Fist do some gentle cardio to bring your heart rate down. Think walking slowly around your living room or doing gentle high knees. Then stretch.

## Sample homebody workout 2

After a gentle five-minute warm-up, try this pyramid set of jumping jacks and step-runs. (Step-runs: Step up and down on the bottom stair quickly with each leg for the required number of repetitions.) Do five jumping jacks, five step-runs, ten jumping jacks, ten step-runs, fifteen jumping jacks, fifteen step-runs, twenty jumping jacks, twenty step-runs, fifteen jumping jacks, fifteen step-runs, ten jumping jacks, ten step-runs, five jumping jacks, and five step-runs. Repeat the entire cycle once. As you gain fitness and stamina, feel free to gradually build up your reps. Make your eventual aim to complete the entire sequence twice.

Strength train three times per week. There are various inexpensive pieces of equipment you can buy for your home including a resistance band, a stability ball, and free weights. See chapter 1 for more equipment options and chapter 10 for additional sample strength workouts.

## Sample at-home full-body workout: "Minutes"

**Warm-up:** Dance or walk up and down the stairs for five minutes.
**Main set:** Pick five strength exercises and two core exercises. Do one minute each of five different strength exercises. Then do one minute each of two different core exercises, and finally two minutes of running up and down your stairs. Rest for one minute. That whole set equals ten minutes. Repeat the set two to three times through. Below is a sample workout. In two to four weeks, when you are bored with this sample circuit, keep the same format, but substitute different exercises. For the strength exercises, continue to prioritize multi-joint strength exercises. In this initial circuit I included step-ups, push-ups, rows, lunges, and monster walks. Other excellent multi-joint exercises are deadlifts, squats, single-arm bench rows, and walking lunges.

## Sample circuit

**Minute I.**

Step-ups: Stand facing a sturdy, hard chair. Place your entire right foot on the chair. Engage your bum to step up. Slowly lower yourself down and repeat ten times. Switch feet and repeat on the opposite side.

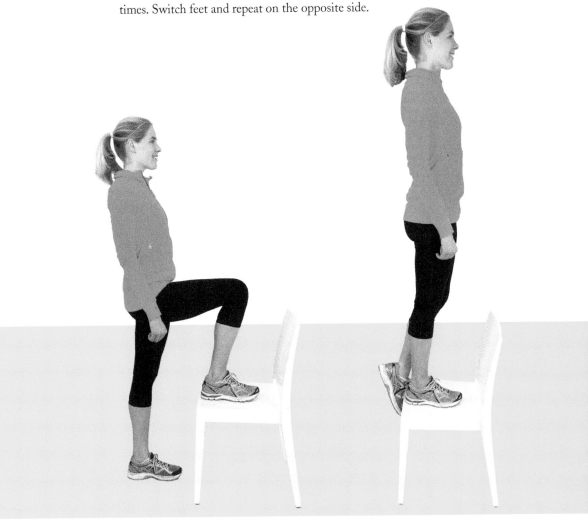

## Minute 2.

➧ Push-ups: Place your hands on the floor feet on the ground. Make sure your bum and core are engaged as you lower yourself down and then raise yourself back up. Your lower back shouldn't be arched or rounded. To modify, do push-ups with your hands on the edge of the sofa or a countertop — so your body is on an incline — or do push-ups with your knees and hands on the floor.

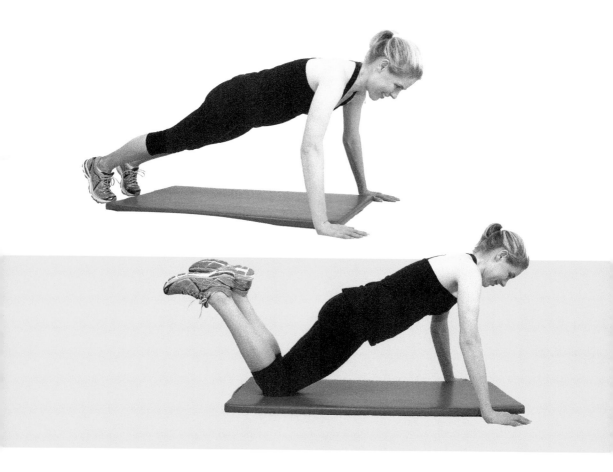

## Minute 3.

➡ Band rows: Attach the band to something at chest height (like a bed post or railing) or latch it into a door frame using a door-frame attachment. Door frame attachments are roughly five dollars and allow you to safely hook the band anywhere into the door frame. Step away from the attachment so that the band has no slack and your arms are straight. Use your shoulder blades to pull your elbows back until your hands are roughly beside your chest. Imagine that you are cracking a walnut with your shoulder blades. Slowly straighten your arms. Control the band — don't let the band control you.

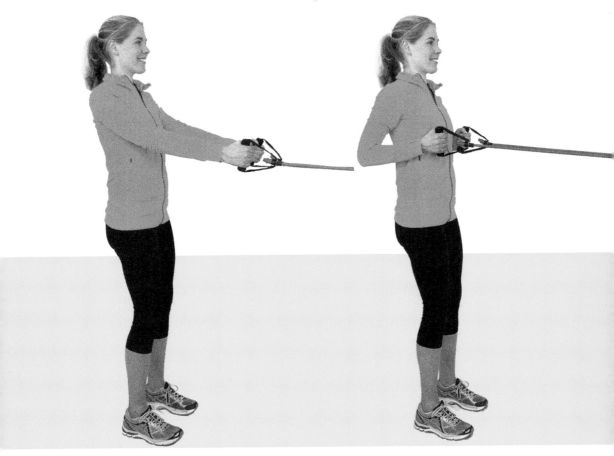

### Minute 4.

⟶ Lunge: Start standing with your feet hip-distance apart. Step your right leg backward into a lunge. Both feet should stay facing forward. Bend both knees so that your body moves toward the floor, then engage the bum muscle of your front leg to stand up. Switch and repeat, with your left leg stepping backward. Start with your arms by your side, no weights. Once you have mastered the form, hold free weights. You can either hold the weights at chest height, elbows bent. Or you can hold the weights by your side, arms straight.

### Minute 5.

⟶ Monster walks: Stand on a resistance band. Hold one end of the band in each hand, feet hip-distance apart. Engage your left bum muscles to step your left leg out to the side. The size of the step is not what is important — think quality. Use your bum, not your foot to push the band out. Bring your right leg toward your left and continue to walk left for thirty seconds. Reverse direction, going right.

### Core exercise I.

⟶ Front plank: Place your forearms and either your knees or the tips of your toes on the ground. Make sure that your bum is not up in the air, your upper back is not rounded, and your lower back is not arched. Your body should look like a plank. If you can easily do a minute from your knees, do the exercise from your toes.

Core exercise 2.

➡ Side plank: Start by lying on your side. Lift up and balance on one forearm and either your knees or the outside edge of your foot. Keep your core engaged. Draw your top shoulder backward and make sure your rib cage is not jutting forward. It should be in-line with your pelvis. If you can easily hold the position for a minute on your knees, do the exercise from the outside edge of your foot.

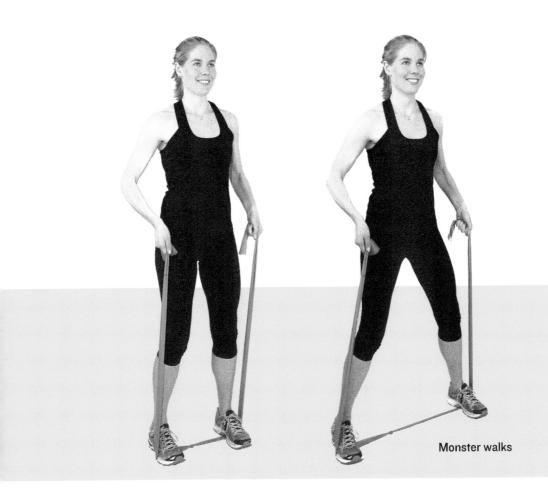

Monster walks

# CHAPTER TAKE-AWAY

Whatever your exercise personality, and regardless of what you do at the gym, aim to take roughly 10,000 steps a day in addition to any structured workouts. Try to sit less and move more in your daily life — don't let yourself off the "steps hook" if you walk or run daily. For more information on how to get your steps, see chapter 3.

Keep in mind that adopting a healthier lifestyle is a process. Your exercise personality is likely to evolve over time; part of the health process is regularly assessing your progress and tweaking your recipe for success. For example, if you are self-conscious now, and therefore a homebody personality, you might develop a love of the gym as you become more body-confident. Fantastic! I encourage you to actively evolve. (There is that word again — actively.) If you develop a program that doesn't work, or if you get bored, don't give up. Assess what the problems are, learn from them, and then create an improved recipe.

Remember, your health quest is something you are doing for YOU! Adopting a healthier lifestyle is about self-care. Care enough about yourself to consume healthy food and make movement a priority.

Learning to understand your established habits and triggers might be complicated and intense, and figuring out how to give yourself the care you deserve will probably be a lengthy process, but the process is worth it. Stay motivated, involved, and dedicated for the long haul. Learn from your health history. Persevere.

# CONCLUSION

ongratulations — you have finished the book. I am so proud of you! If you are thinking "I read this, but now what?" remind yourself that when it comes to adopting a healthier lifestyle, getting started is often more than half the battle. Simply buying and reading the book counts as getting started — you have accumulated a number of drops in your health bucket. Now it is time to capitalize on your positive momentum. Let this book be your positive catalyst for change.

Digesting the information from this book and incorporating it into your life might take you a while — that is to be expected. Anything worth doing takes mindfulness and perseverance — and almost nothing is more important than your health. Initially it will take you conscious effort to change your lifestyle; but if you stick with it, gradually your preferences will change; making healthier choices will slowly seem more natural. Remember, adopting a healthier lifestyle is all about trending positive. Instead of aiming for health perfection, which most of us have probably tried in the past, aim to have more healthy habits this month than you did last month.

When you fall off your health horse, don't be discouraged. We all fall off once in a while — expect setbacks and then learn from them. Don't allow that one less-than-ideal choice to spiral into multiple unhealthy choices. Instead, get back on your health horse a more informed rider. Learn from your unhealthy choice. Did you make the choice because you let yourself get too hungry? Were you emotionally eating? Did you not take the time to set yourself up for success? Maybe you need to set out your exercise clothes the night before and/or schedule your workouts into your calendar. Whatever the case, make a mental note of what went wrong so you can proactively avoid those situations in the future. Whatever you do, don't get discouraged or feel guilty, those emotions are counterproductive. Your unhealthy habits were not formed in a day, so your healthy habits will not materialize overnight.

Plus, the realities of your life will change, and as they do your goals and health expectations should also evolve. If you get a new job, move to a new city, or have a child your life rhythms will change — actively assess your new rhythms and plan accordingly. For example, I have gone through this "rejigging" process with all my clients who become moms; they had to completely rework their workout plans and expectations. At first they were overwhelmed trying to fit in work, having a child, and training. They felt they couldn't do anything well enough. What I told them is that negotiating any new situation takes courage and determination. You're going to miss a few workouts — expect that

with any large lifestyle change. Instead of getting discouraged, be proud that you are not simply giving up. Actively assess the new situation, then adapt and grow. All of these clients have found different ways to negotiate their new lives. Some work out on their lunch break. Others train when their children are in bed. Some no longer belong to a gym and simply train at home. All of these are great options. The main take-away is that they were successful not because they were perfect immediately, but because they took the time to assess their situation and form realistic goals. They actively took control of their own health.

You can also take control of your own health — I know you can! Start to look for opportunities to be active. Get yourself a pedometer, walk at lunch with a colleague, go on active dates with your partner, play sports with your kids, and take the stairs. Never forget that adopting a healthier lifestyle is an active process! Love yourself enough to consciously plan your diet and your movement patterns. Your health choices add up. What you eat and how you move today becomes your body tomorrow. Your body's tissues are in a constant state of renewal; the cells that line your stomach are replaced every five days, red blood cells last only four months, and the cells in your liver are replaced every 300 to 500 days. Even your bones are not permanent; your entire skeleton renews itself roughly every ten years. Your body is always evolving. Your health is not a finite goal; adopting a healthier lifestyle and maintaining a healthy weight is a life-long, ever-evolving process.

Adopting a healthier lifestyle is about self-care, and it is a privilege. It is easy to forget that eating well and exercising are things we are doing for ourselves, not to ourselves. Too often health is framed as deprivation — something you have to do rather than something you want to do, an existence based on the cake you can't eat and the social activity (such as drinking) you have to cut out. It is no wonder so many of us yo-yo diet and exercise, develop feelings of rebellion toward healthy food and exercise, and adopt the all-too-common "I deserve" mentality. Who wants to feel constrained and deprived? Break this cycle by reframing your concept of health. Instead of understanding health as all the things you have to give up, adopt what I call the "find your kiwi" approach. A kiwi represents something healthy that you truly love — or at least something healthy that you don't despise. Find things you are genuinely excited to eat or do. Do you like to garden, walk with friends, or play a sport? If so, build those modes of exercise into your life. Do you like fresh berries or sweet potatoes? If so, make sure to include those in your weekly diet.

This approach stemmed from a conversation I had with a client. She was no longer motivated to stick to her plan because eating healthy and exercising had become just another thing on her to-do list. Her homework was to come up with two healthy things that she genuinely would be excited to eat or do. She decided she enjoyed kiwis (but never bought them because her family didn't like them) and gardening. I told her that whenever she wanted junk food she should instead have a kiwi (or another healthy choice worthy of the name kiwi), and whenever she couldn't motivate herself to go to the gym she should garden instead. That way she wouldn't feel constrained or deprived.

Finding your kiwi is about gradually learning to associate healthier choices with positive feelings; you are always more apt to continue a program when it includes foods and activities you like. Put together a list of nutritiously dense yet scrumptious food options and exercise activities that don't feel like a chore. When you find yourself falling into the "Poor me, I can't eat X" or "Poor me, I have to exercise" mentality, instead say, "Which of my yummy kiwis am I lucky enough to eat or do today?"

As you work through your health process, reread the chapters as needed. I designed the book with the hope that you would be able to pick it up and read sections whenever you need an extra bit of pep in your step. Go back and reread sections when you need extra motivation or when you want to refresh your memory. Explore suggestions that you haven't tried yet. If you don't know which chapter to go back to, or which Kathleenism to implement first, start with these four suggestions. Out of everything I have written in this book, these are the four strategies that work best for me.

1. Use my ten-minute rule. When I don't want to exercise, I tell myself I have to do something for at least ten minutes. Anyone can do anything for ten minutes. I tell myself that if after ten minutes I want to stop, I can. At least I have done something. But whenever I start, I always just end up doing a full workout — getting started is always the hardest part.

2. Have a health mantra. When I don't want to train, I tell myself, "Kathleen, the worse you feel the more important your workout is! You will feel better if you move. The options are sweat or regret. Just do something." If this mantra doesn't resonate with you, make up your own. Repeat it out loud whenever you want to skip a workout.

3. Ask what your future self would want you to do. If I want chocolate cake or to skip a workout, I try to put myself in the future. I aim to make my current decision based on what future Kathleen will feel proud of.

4. Remember that being able to move and eat well is a privilege. I am lucky enough that I can buy yummy berries and that my body is healthy enough to move. I consciously work to flip my mindset around health. I aim to find the positive and appreciate my health privilege. Don't focus on what you can't have or do. Focus on what you are lucky enough to be able to have or do.

Consider giving a friend or colleague the book so you have someone to discuss the ideas with. Think about asking that person to become your fitness buddy; try a few of the workouts from the book with them or make a date to go to a fun fitness class. I always enjoy meeting a friend for a class. Many of my clients who are the most successful are successful because they have a buddy. I have a few mother-daughter teams that train together, as well as husbands and wives who come and train together. Both sets of teams love spending the hour with each other, and I know they also feel it is helpful to have a loved one going through the same process with them.

Any time you need some extra motivation, find me on my social media sites. My website, which I update regularly, is kathleentrotter.com. Follow me on Twitter (@ KTrotterFitness) or find me on Facebook (www.facebook.com/KathleenTrotter) or

Pinterest (www.pinterest.com/KTrotter Fitness). I also have a monthly newsletter, which you can sign up for on my website. The newsletter is full of healthy recipes, fun exercises, and interesting articles.

If you remember one word from this book it should be "persevere." Your health is not a finite goal. It is not a battle that needs to be won. Battles end — your health process does not. You simply have to resolve to persevere and aim to trend positive.

It takes time to change your taste buds and your habits. Learning to love healthy food and movement is a process — I have not always loved running, but now it is my bliss. Embrace how lucky you are to have the power to make healthy choices. Trust me, if you persevere, over time your preferences will change, your list of kiwis will grow, and you will slowly begin to gravitate more naturally toward healthier options.

Don't let yourself fall into the common trap of believing that finding the "perfect" diet will ensure that you will reach your health and fitness goals. An intelligent plan can be a helpful jumping off point, but if you don't change your mindset you will simply continue to fall off your health horse or find the loopholes in every plan you follow.

You can become the fit version of yourself you want to be. I know you can. Ultimately, being successful is not about the plan you choose to follow; a plan can only work if you have a healthy and productive mindset. Don't transfer responsibility for your health onto any one plan. Take charge of your own health journey.

Once you start to trend positive you will feel better physically, emotionally, and mentally, and feeling better will help to propel you forward. I have evolved — with conscious, active effort — into a different version of Kathleen than I was in high school. I am more self-confident, I have more energy, I am more positive, and I am physically and mentally stronger.

Your health process starts today. Get up and go for a walk. Remember, every drop in your bucket counts.

# ACKNOWLEDGEMENTS

I consider myself one of the luckiest women in the world; I have so many supportive and emotionally generous people in my life. Without them I would never have been able to write this book.

First and foremost, I want to thank my mother, Kate, for helping me become the person I am today. Not only does my mother offer unwavering emotional and financial support, she models the type of human being I am working to become. I only hope one day to be half the woman she is.

James Harnum and family, who initially pushed me to write the book, come a close second. I only decided to put together the proposal after numerous family dinners where I was told I absolutely could succeed. Specifically, thank you Bill Harnum for walking me through how to put together a proposal and get an agent, and thank you James Harnum for your unwavering support through the entire process. James, you helped me become the writer I am today, and I will always be grateful.

It is my pleasure to thank my second family, Clay, Harriet, Emma, and Kate. Living with you taught me to speak up and be proud of my opinions. Without all of you in my life I would never have had the courage to write anything, let alone a book!

I also want to thank all of my friends, specifically the four who had a quantifiable impact on this project. Kathryn, thank you for helping me through the entire editing process. Without your help Dundurn would have received a manuscript riddled with typos. Julie, Jack, and Emily, thank you for your support and for helping me brainstorm titles for the book. Emily, you in particular deserve a shout out. You are one outstanding friend. Bouncing ideas off you helped me to frame the book. Specifically, thank you for inspiring the "choose your own adventure" theme of the final chapter, and for helping me craft the "market analysis" for my original proposal.

I also want to thank a number of individuals who have mentored me along the way and/or had a positive effect on my career. Thank you Samantha at the Metro Central YMCA for teaching me how to be an aerobics instructor. Thank you to everyone at Trainers Fitness for giving me my start as a trainer. Thank you Kirsten for encouraging me to spread my wings, leave Trainers, and work at a boutique studio. Kirsten, I always wanted to "be you." Thank you to Rasha and Maureen for believing in

my writing and helping me get started as a writer, and to everyone at Flaman Fitness for outfitting my studio so nicely and always being so supportive — especially Eric.

I have such amazing family, friends, colleagues, and clients — I can't possibly name them all. A few who need to be mentioned are Adam, my dad, my wonderful sister Trisanna, Reva, Andrea, Judith, Alison and Bill, Kelly and Mel, Tanya and Mia, Laura, Harry, Isa, Jenny and Julio, Sammy, Karen, Ron (my first personal training client ever), Judith, Carol, Trixie and Danny, Marvin and Miriam, Krista, Louise, Tari, Linda, my godmother Maureen, Tara, my web designer Tracy, Ashleigh Goodbody, everyone at Quesada, and my incredible assistant Angeliqua, who helps me keep my studio clean and who I couldn't live without.

Last, my thank-you list wouldn't be complete without a shout out to my amazing agent Jesse and the publishing team at Dundurn. Thank you for having faith in my vision.

# ABOUT THE AUTHOR

Kathleen Trotter has been a personal trainer and Pilates specialist for almost fifteen years, and a fitness writer and media expert for seven. For the past five years, she has been the featured personal trainer in the *Globe and Mail's* online *Fitness Basic* video series. She also writes two columns for the *Globe and Mail* and blogs regularly for *The Huffington Post*; has written for *Impact Magazine, Healthy Directions* magazine, *Breathe, Alive, Canadian Running, Today's Parent, Chatelaine,* and *Glow;* and is often quoted in other publications such as the *Toronto Star* and *Toronto Sun.* Kathleen makes regular TV and media appearances on *CTV News, CHCH News, Breakfast Television,* and the CBC. She has been a guest on the radio shows *Beyond the Cheers* and *The John Oakley Show.* She is the health ambassador for the Quesada chain of restaurants, for whom she provides "Trotter Tips" and advocates healthy nutrition choices on the go. She also has the pleasure of blogging for and working closely with Flaman Fitness.

In May 2015, Kathleen opened a private, boutique personal training studio in downtown Toronto. She was voted one of Toronto's top 10 personal trainers by BlogTo.

Kathleen has not always lived an active and healthy lifestyle. In fact, she became a personal trainer because exercise literally changed her life. In her early teens Kathleen was overweight and had low self-esteem. That all changed when she was given a membership to the YMCA as a grade-eight graduation gift. She started to run and lift weights, and soon the girl who would do anything to get out of gym class was running marathons, lifting weights, and playing on basketball and baseball teams. Kathleen feels that changing her lifestyle was the best thing that she ever did; she became a personal trainer to help others form healthier habits. She truly believes that exercise has the ability to energize and exhilarate, and that if your workouts are making you feel worse about yourself, then you are doing something wrong!

Kathleen holds a master's degree from the University of Toronto and is currently working to graduate from the Canadian School of Natural Nutrition. Find out more about Kathleen and sign up for her monthly newsletter on her website: kathleentrotter.com. Follow her at www.facebook.com/KathleenTrotter, @KTrotterFitness on Twitter and Pinterest, and kathleentrotterfitness on Instagram.

## Image Credits

6......Malina Kaija
10......kosmosIII, iStock
13......Kanawa_Studio, iStock
15......Malina Kaija
24......Jennifer Powers
25......Jennifer Powers
26......Jennifer Powers
27......Jennifer Powers
36......mihailomilovanovic, iStock
37......miflippo, iStock
42......Rüstem GÜRLER, iStock
45......Dirima, iStock
64......izf, iStock
70......pixdeluxe, iStock
74......Martinina, iStock
79......izf, iStock
82......Maximkostenko, iStock
84......Tuned_In, iStock

85......progressman, Shutterstock
90......jonas unruh, iStock
94......Sarsmis, iStock
95......sf_foodphoto, iStock
100......Dragon Images, Shutterstock
109......Christopher Futcher, iStock
112......Julia Nichols, iStock
118......izf, iStock
136......Christopher Futcher, iStock
140......Neustockimages, iStock
143......Jennifer Powers
147......Jennifer Powers
149......Jennifer Powers
155......Jennifer Powers
156......Jennifer Powers
157......Jennifer Powers
158......Jennifer Powers
159......Jennifer Powers

160......Jennifer Powers
161......Jennifer Powers
162......Jennifer Powers
163......Jennifer Powers
164......Jennifer Powers
165......Jennifer Powers
166......Jennifer Powers
167......wundervisuals, iStock
169......Jennifer Powers
170......Jennifer Powers
171......Jennifer Powers
172......Jennifer Powers
173......Jennifer Powers
174......Jennifer Powers
177......Jennifer Powers
178......Jennifer Powers
179......Jennifer Powers
181......Jennifer Powers